EXPLORATIONS IN
CHICANO
PSYCHOLOGY

EXPLORATIONS IN
CHICANO
PSYCHOLOGY

Edited by
Augustine Barón, Jr.

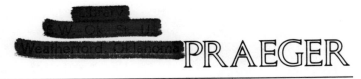

PRAEGER

PRAEGER SPECIAL STUDIES • PRAEGER SCIENTIFIC

Library of Congress Cataloging in Publication Data

Barón, Augustine.
  Explorations in Chicano psychology.

  Includes indexes.
  1. Mexican Americans--Psychology. 2. Mexican
Americans--Mental health services. I. Title. [DNLM:
1. Hispanic Americans--Psychology. 2. Mental health
services--United States. GN 270 B265e]
RC451.5.M48B36   155.8'46872073   81-2639
ISBN 0-03-058016-1   AACR2

Published in 1981 by Praeger Publishers
CBS Educational and Professional Publishing
A Division of CBS, Inc.
521 Fifth Avenue, New York, New York 10175 U.S.A.

© 1981 by Praeger Publishers

123456789   145   987654321

Printed in the United States of America

To

Floyd H. Martínez

and

Amado M. Padilla

in recognition of their contributions to
the advancement of Chicano Psychology

PREFACE

Looking retrospectively at the developmental phases of this book, I can project myself back to a time that now seems long ago and far away. Actually, the prospectus for the work began the Spring of 1978 when I gathered together a group of Chicano graduate students of the University of Texas at Austin and formed an "ad hoc advisory board." Their enthusiasm was contagious and it spurred me on to develop a suitable outline. Several of those students have since received their doctorates and also have contributed chapters to this book.

In the early phases of promoting the prospectus to potential publishers, the idea met with mixed reactions. It became clear that a volume in a new area like Chicano psychology would have a cool reception in a competitive trade like the publishing business. Also, the hesitancies, I believe, are characteristic of the process of "nudging" a subspecialty into established, mainstream academia. Thus, Chicano psychology has its battles to fight in establishing itself as a legitimate specialty in the field of psychology. The publication of this book and others like it will strengthen such efforts.

I chose the title Explorations in Chicano Psychology to convey a sense of this area's nascent stage of development. We are just beginning to explore the vast frontiers of Chicano psychology. Thus, the reader can consider the chapters in this book as preliminary "scouting reports." Overall, the volume is divided into three major branches of psychology that I felt would capture the main lines of research interest. While not all avenues of investigation are represented, it is hoped that the ten chapters presented here will convey the state of knowledge in several key areas.

Part I, Community and Social Psychology, contains four chapters each reviewing and synthesizing the current state of knowledge in their respective topic areas. Oscar Ramírez and Carlos H. Árce present a detailed, "stereotype-busting" chapter on the Chicano family. By carefully analyzing available data, the heterogeneity of Chicano families emerges, while emphasizing undergirding strengths. Frank Cota-Robles Newton, working with the meager research literature available, summarizes our current knowledge of the Hispanic elderly and points to research questions much deserving of attention. Melba J. T. Vásquez

and Anna M. González focus their attention on sex-role stereotyping among Chicanos. Traditional views are juxtaposed with
current research and theory, which gives rise to new conclusions
about feminine and masculine role behaviors. The last chapter
in this section discusses what I consider to be the "cornerstone
construct" for Chicano psychology, namely, acculturation.
Richard H. Mendoza and Joe L. Martínez present a sophisticated
elaboration of this important construct and relate their discussion
to its heuristic value in psychological research.

Part II, Counseling and Educational Psychology, presents
three chapters, each concerned with a different aspect of the
educational process. Edward T. Rincón's chapter discusses
the role of aptitude tests in influencing the participation of
minorities in higher education. The validity of such tests is
examined along with specific factors that may affect performance.
Moving from testing to admissions selection procedures, Jude
Valdez summarizes the major issues faced by colleges and universities and the different models that can be employed to provide
flexible admissions procedures. The last chapter examines
minority college students' characteristics and concerns after
they have already entered school. Melba J. T. Vásquez, Jude
Valdez, and I discuss findings from two separate studies at two
different university campuses employing a comparable survey
instrument.

The topic area in Chicano psychology that has received
the greatest attention within the last two decades is mental health
and all its related aspects. Part III, Mental Health: Issues and
Research, contains three chapters, two of which are timely
research reports. The first chapter in this part tackles the
prevailing conclusions regarding research on the utilization of
mental health services by Chicanos. By carefully examining
methodological flaws in the literature, Steven López argues for
differing conclusions from those commonly gleaned by past researchers. Israel Cuéllar, Lorwen C. Harris, and Nancy Naron
present the results of a ground-breaking research project. They
discuss data related to the evaluation of an innovative culture-
modulated treatment milieu for psychotic Chicano inpatients.
Finally, A. Patrícia Mendoza presents findings from her study
of stress and coping patterns among Anglo and Chicano university
students. The study combined the latest theory and methodology
in an attempt to expand upon validity and reliability considerations in the measurement of stress and coping responses.

In closing, I would like to express my appreciation to
numerous individuals who have helped both directly and indirectly
in the production of this book. Foremostly, the 14 contributors

deserve my gratitude for undertaking the onerous task of writing chapters specifically for this volume. Each member of my ad hoc advisory board also deserves my thanks: Anna González, Joe Lerma, Chris Lovato, Patrícia Mendoza, Edward Rincón, and Melba Vásquez. I take great pride and pleasure in knowing that four of these people (González, Mendoza, Rincón, and Vásquez) have contributed chapters as well.

The pragmatics of producing a book depend on the invaluable skills of secretaries. I have been blessed with two generous individuals, Deborah Rice and Mitzi Barrow, who accommodated readily to the ever-escalating demands of my editorial obsessions. The unsavory task of indexing was enthusiastically aided by Richard Cohen, whose infectious humor came at just the right moments. To David Drum, James Clack, and Marilyn Alexander, the director, associate director, and executive assistant respectively of the Counseling-Psychological Services Center at the University of Texas at Austin, I express my thanks for providing administrative support for the completion of this work.

No book can be born without a publisher and so I convey my gratitude to Praeger Publishers and my editor, George Zimmar, for consenting to print this work, thereby making it accessible to a wider audience.

AUGUSTINE BARÓN, JR.

CONTENTS

LIST OF TABLES AND FIGURES

PART I
COMMUNITY AND SOCIAL PSYCHOLOGY

1

THE CONTEMPORARY CHICANO FAMILY: AN EMPIRICALLY BASED REVIEW

Oscar Ramírez and Carlos H. Árce

Both the volume and the orientation of recent writings on Chicano family life have closely paralleled the rapidly growing overall body of literature on or by Chicanos. Although some important theoretical expositions based on empirical research on the Chicano have been produced in sociology and history, there is a very serious neglect of empirical work in sociopsychological research on Chicanos. Few areas have been empirically ignored as consistently as the Chicano family.

The literature on la familia (the family) falls into four broad types: first, an older, often flawed literature that is based mostly on observational field research and occasional local surveys in traditional enclaves of the Mexican population, and that attributes a pathological, detrimental character and role to the family; second, a reactive literature, mostly by Chicanos, intended to counter the former, but often presenting an idealized, romanticized, and empirically unsupported characterization of the family; third, a modest but rapidly proliferating number of articles and dissertations that are focused, data based, and more rigorous in design and conceptualization; and fourth, several "review" articles that periodically attempt, with mixed success, to integrate the existent literature on the family. This chapter seeks to fill an important void by providing a current review that focuses exclusively on the state of empirically based knowledge about la familia.

This review differs from others in two important ways. First, it comes soon after the appearance of important new research contributions on Chicano family phenomena. More importantly, the chapter is guided principally by the need to bring clarity to prominent family issues, such as the composition, form, and structure of the family, intrafamilial exchange relations, and familial roles, which have often been, and still are, the

3

source of much conceptual confusion and distortion in the larger body of literature on Chicano families. Recent empirical work, mostly by Chicano scholars, in each of the areas covered in this chapter significantly expands our understanding of the contemporary Chicano family and merits this new integrative assessment.

A DEMOGRAPHIC PROFILE

Before reviewing the behavioral science research on substantive issues regarding family, it is valuable to consider the demographic characteristics of Chicano families, and to use them as an objective backdrop against which to examine the actual studies of significant aspects of family life. The principal source of information for this brief profile is census data, particularly in the 1970 U.S. Census of Population and annual Current Population Surveys for March and June.[1] As far as possible, this profile is both diachronic, pointing out patterns across time, and comparative, contrasting Chicano families to other populations in the United States.

Composition and Size

As of March 1979, over 1.5 million families were headed by persons of Mexican origin. This number is about 65 percent larger than the number of Mexican-origin families reported by the 1970 census. Although population growth due to new births, increased life expectancy, and both legal and undocumented immigration has been substantial, this increment is as much a function of the Census Bureau's improved ability to enumerate Chicanos as it is of actual population increases. The size of Chicano families, as measured by the number of persons per family, has gradually decreased over the past decade, declining from slightly over 4.5 to just over 4 persons per family. However, Chicano family size has consistently remained at least 25 percent greater than non-Chicano family size. The fact that relatively large families remain a significant phenomenon for Chicanos is demonstrated by the proportion of large families defined as those with 6 or more persons. About 21 percent of all Chicano families are this large, in contrast to 13 percent for Puerto Rican families, 17 percent for Blacks, and only 8 percent for Whites.

Chicanos are also younger than other groups. Their median age is about 21 years below the median age for the U.S.

population. Fourteen percent of Chicanos are under five years old, while only 7.6 percent of the total population is that young. By contrast, when one looks at the other end of the age spectrum, only 4.5 percent of all Chicanos are 65 years old and over, against 10.7 percent of the total population. From a family unit perspective, only 6 percent of Chicano families are headed by persons over the age of 65 years, against 15 percent for non-Chicano families.

Conversely, the presence of minor children (under age 18) is a more frequent occurrence in Chicano families. Non-Chicano families have a mean of two minor children in the home per family, while Chicanos have three. While only 54 percent of all non-Chicano families have children under 18 years of age at home, over 76 percent of Chicano families do. Similarly, Chicano households are more likely than non-Chicano households to have relatives other than spouse or child present. There are 23 such "other" relatives per 100 Chicano households, versus only 11 per 100 in the total population.

Although the concept of family head with its automatic assignation of the male as the head of husband-wife families has become less appropriate and relevant, in light of families with working spouses or multifamily households, it still has some utility, especially for consideration of female-headed families. About one of every six (16.1 percent) Chicano families is maintained by a woman, in comparison to 13.5 percent of non-Chicano families. The Chicano family in this regard is much closer to the White norm (11 percent) than to the Black (35 percent) or Puerto Rican (37 percent).

In summary, compared to other populations in the United States, Chicano families are larger, have younger family heads, and more minor children and other relatives in the home than all other racial ethnic groups, and they are significantly less likely to be female-headed than are Black or Puerto Rican families.

Marriage Patterns

The Mexican origin population does not differ significantly from the total population in regard to marital status. For the population 14 years old and over, Chicano men are slightly more likely to be single (33 percent) and less likely to be married (62 percent) than for the total population (30 percent and 64 percent respectively). For Chicanas, 28 percent are single, versus 23 percent for the total population. There is no difference in the proportion married between Chicanas and other women.

However, sizable and important differences do appear when one examines age at marriage. In the 18- and 19-year-old cohort, over 40 percent of all Chicanas have married, in contrast to 25 percent for other Hispanic women, 23 percent for White women, and 12 percent for Black women. Although the differences are not as pronounced, Chicano men also marry at a younger age than Black, White, or other Hispanic men. In short, Chicano families are formed earlier in the life span and children are born at a younger stage in their parents' lives and in larger numbers than for other racial/ethnic groups.

The incidence of marital breakup is slightly more frequent for Chicanos than for the White population, but considerably less frequent than for other minority groups, namely Blacks and other Hispanics. The proportions of men 14 years old and over who are either divorced or separated are 11.7 percent for Blacks, 7.3 percent for other Hispanics, 6.8 percent for Chicanos and 5.9 percent for Whites. For women, the figures are 19.1 percent for Blacks, 16.6 percent for other Hispanics, 10.7 percent for Chicanas, and 8.0 percent for White women. Other data suggest that the divorce rates for Chicanos and other Hispanics are actually lower than for Whites and that the rates are as much an artifact of reduced rates of remarriage and longer periods before remarriage.

A further marital indicator especially relevant to the study of cultural maintenance and assimilation is the rate of endogamy. Current population survey data for the past few years suggests that the proportions of Chicanos married within the ethnic group are very close for males and females (about 85 percent of those married), with Chicanas slightly more likely to have non-Chicano husbands than Chicanos having non-Chicana wives. Further, the statistics for the past several years suggest a remarkably steady rate of ethnic intermarriage, with a small but nonsignificant trend toward less intermarriage overall with some regional differences. In regard to the salience of extended family ties, low rates of intermarriage may be associated with a familistic orientation.

Fertility and Childbearing

As has happened with women in other ethnic groups, the childbearing rates for Chicanas appear to have declined over the past decade. However, fully acceptable data are not available, and we have here relied upon overall Hispanic data, extrapolating from it for the greater fertility of Chicanas compared to other

Hispanic women. Lifetime births expected (births to date plus
future births expected) per 1,000 women, 18 to 34 years old,
are 2,114 for Whites, 2,267 for Blacks, and 2,390 for Hispanics.
Accepting the Chicano versus other Hispanic differences reported
elsewhere, one can safely assume a figure of at least 2,600 per
1,000 Chicanas. Unlike Black or White women, Chicanas with
some college education expect more children than those who are
only high school graduates but have not attended college. This
suggests that the Chicano culture's proclivity for higher fertility
and large families resists the otherwise strong and deflating
impact of higher education. However, evidence of declining
future fertility is found in data showing that younger Chicanas
(18 to 24 year olds) expect fewer lifetime births than a Chicana
cohort a decade older (30 to 34 year olds). The difference between age cohorts is also more pronounced for Chicanas than
for either Blacks or Whites, thus suggesting a larger relative
decline in fertility.

Socioeconomic Factors

The median income in 1976 of Chicano families ($10,000)
was significantly lower than the median family income for White
families ($16,000), but was higher than family income of Puerto
Ricans ($7,700) or Blacks ($9,045). As would be expected,
given women's overall smaller share in earned income, median
income for female-headed Chicano families was less than half
that of male-headed Chicano families ($5,559 versus $11,270).
Median income of husband-wife families, with both in the paid
labor force, was $14,194. Larger families suffer the burden of
low income more severely. Chicano families with four children
have lower median total incomes than Chicano families with fewer
or no children. Chicano families below the poverty level in 1976
were larger than Chicano families overall (mean of 4.52 persons
versus 4.26), were more likely to be headed by females (37 percent versus 16 percent), and were more likely to be headed by
someone not a high school graduate (73 percent versus 57 percent).
The participation of Chicanas in the paid labor force is
another demographic indicator of much relevance to any study
of family life. The rate of labor force participation for Chicanas
has increased steadily from about 30 percent in 1970 to over
45 percent in 1977. The present participation rate is now nearly
at the level of the total female population. The major area of
employment for Chicanas is in the operative sector. This dramatic

change is almost certain to have, or to be having already, an impact of major proportions on the functioning of the Chicano family on many levels. In a subsequent chapter, we discuss this issue in more detail.

This brief demographic profile attempts to obviate the simplistic and stereotypic characterization of the Chicano family. On some dimensions, Chicano families appear similar to other ethnic/racial groups, on other dimensions, Chicanos differ substantially and dramatically from the same groups. Sometimes Chicano families cluster closely, in a statistical sense, with other Hispanic groups but just as often, on other traits, Chicanos are more similar to non-Hispanic populations than to other Hispanic groups. The contrasts and similarities between Chicanos and other groups are sometimes predictable and explainable, at other times unexplained, surprising, and unresearched and at still other times subtle and undramatic. This profile emphasizes the reality of demographic diversity and range of Chicano families Yet the profile also sharply identifies and demonstrates the distinctive features of Chicano families in terms of tendencies regarding size, growth, age, composition, extendedness, and economic status.

REFORMULATIONS AND RECENT EMPIRICAL WORK

As suggested earlier, a great deal of conceptual reformulation has appeared in the literature on the nature and functions of contemporary Chicano families. Guided by the priority we have given to empirical research findings, we have organized the literature into five topics, each representing an aspect of Chicano family life. Our choice of these five aspects is founded on the joint existence of stereotypic characterizations and recent empirical research about each of them, producing lively debates. The five topics are: the structure and functions of Chicano families; the nature of exchange relationships among family members; family and gender roles; conjugal decision making among Chicano couples; and a reexamination of the concept of machismo.

Structure and Functions of Chicano Families

A fundamental focus of research and reformulation that provides an anchor for empirical explorations of familial phenomen is the structure of the family and its effect on the norms and behaviors of its members. Two related but historically independent debates have intersected in the recent literature on the nature of the Mexican-American family: the relative value and utility of the nuclear versus the extended family in contemporary society, and the validity of the trigenerational household model of the extended family for depicting the prevailing family structure among Chicanos.

The aspects of Chicano family life of most interest and relevance both in the above debates and in the present review are familism, both as a set of norms or values and as behavioral patterns of Chicanos, and the extended family system, involving relatively strong and extensive bonds with kin beyond the nuclear family. Like other concepts of fundamental importance to an understanding of Chicano life, "familism" and "extended family system" are inconsistently and confusingly treated in the literature. We view familism as a multidimensional concept that incorporates distinct aspects involving structure, behavior, norms and attitudes, and social identity, each of which requires separate measurement and analytic treatment (Árce, 1978). The central dimensions, normative and behavioral familism, are values and behaviors reflecting the importance of the family for the individual as well as the relative emphasis and priority given to the needs of aggregate units (families) as opposed to individual and personal needs. The extended family system, as a concrete manifestation of a familistic orientation, refers to that network of relatives including grandparents, aunts, and uncles, married sisters and brothers and their children, and also compadres (coparents) and padrinos (godparents) with whom Chicanos actively maintain bonds.

For over 20 years, family scholars have raised substantial theoretical and empirical challenges to the notion that there exists "a basic disharmony between modern democratic industrial society and extended family relations" (Litwak, 1960a, p. 9). Prior to these challenges, the predominant viewpoint was that extended family relations impeded individual mobility while the isolated nuclear family more effectively promoted it. In challenging this, Litwak suggested instead that the modified extended family was not only consonant with mobility but also more functional than the isolated nuclear family: "The modified extended family consists of a series of nuclear families bound together on an equalitarian basis, with a strong emphasis on these extended family bonds as an end value" (1960a, p. 10).

Litwak (1960a, 1960b, and 1965) has found empirical support for the following hypotheses: first, that the extended family, through the provision of aid across class lines, allows the nuclear family, which is occupationally upwardly mobile, to retain its extended kin contacts despite differences in class position, and since this aid is isolated from the occupational system, it does not hinder mobility based on merit (1960a); and second, "that persons separated from their families [retain] their extended family orientation; those with close family identification [are] as likely, if not more likely, to leave their family for occupational reasons; those on the upswing of their careers [are] apt to move away from their families and to receive family support; . . . and that the modified extended family seems to be uniquely suited to provide succor during periods of movement" (1960b, p. 234). There is evidence of pervasive kinship ties in urban centers throughout the world. Repeated findings that point to the importance of kinship ties in instrumental activities of urban dwellers refute the proposition that extended kinship systems are incompatible with the needs of industrial societies (see, for example, Bennett & Despres, 1960). Despite the prevalence of these findings in general family research, the literature on Chicanos, their culture, and family has consistently emphasized the hindering effect of culture and family on the individual.

The second debate is on the accuracy and validity of various models of family structure for depicting the prevailing type of Chicano family today. The major contributor to conceptual work in this area is Sena-Rivera (1973, 1976, 1977, and 1979). Central to Sena-Rivera's research is the premise that the traditional Mexican-American family has been erroneously likened to the classical European extended family. The classical European extended family model is the trigenerational household of children, parents, and grandparents in an interdependent environment. After presenting data that demonstrate the absolute and relative infrequency of trigenerational households in the Chicano population, Sena-Rivera proposes an alternative approach that is more validly applied to the Chicano. His casa-familia model makes a sharp and important distinction between the household (casa) and the kinship network (familia).

In his historical-anthropological examination of the Mexican extended family, Sena (1973) points to the Aztec calpulli as a possible antecedent of the Mexican-American extended family. Existing in an urban, preindustrial setting, the calpulli was a parcel of land shared by independent consanguineous nuclear families living in close proximity to each other. Although the evidence for this direct historical link between contemporary Chicanos and the Aztecs is tenuous, this formal depiction of the extended family is most important. The casa-familia model is basically different in structure from the European trigenerational household model. Sena-Rivera (1976) emphatically states:

The tri-generational household has never been the
norm for Mexico or for Mexicans in the United States
or for other Chicanos, except at times of individual
extended family or conjugal family stress, or periods
of general societal disorganization. Instead, what is
normative and actual is a subjectively compact social
organization unit clustering of essentially independent
nuclear or conjugal households. (pp. 5-6, emphasis
in the original)

The most recent data substantiating his position is Sena-
Rivera's (1977, 1979) intensive study of four trigenerational
Mexican-descent families in the Michigan-Indiana-Illinois region.
The voluminous data gathered from in-depth interviews with
family members spanning three generations served to confirm,
in broad and descriptive terms, the hypothesis that the Chicano
family represents a special case of modified extended or kin-
integrated family, and that the form and structure of the Chicano
extended family did not develop within American industrial society,
but rather transferred from Mexico.

The debate on the structure of the contemporary Chicano
family is important for understanding the family's function and
the extent to which its structure serves its members well. The
evidence for the existence of an extended structure is persuasive
even if there is not consensus on whether the Chicano extended
family is primarily a cultural holdover or primarily a functional
adaptation. While there is insufficient empirical evidence, we
conceptualize the contemporary Chicano extended family chiefly
as a dynamic and adaptive institution. The next empirical question is then whether this structure provides a mechanism of
social/emotional support and whether there are differences in
this regard between Chicanos and other populations.

Recent investigations by Padilla and his colleagues on the
nature of emotional support systems among Chicanos and Anglos
provide the best empirical basis for understanding this function
of the family. These studies are based on survey interviews
of 666 Mexican-Americans and 340 Anglo-Americans in the Southern
California cities of Oxnard, Santa Barbara, and Santa Paula,
where the proportions of Chicanos are 34 percent, 21 percent,
and 41 percent respectively. Given that earlier researchers
(for example Grebler, Moore, & Guzmán, 1970) suggested that
urbanization and acculturation were destroying or undermining
the Chicano extended family, the findings of Keefe, Padilla,
and Carlos (1978a, 1978b, and 1979) in the areas of familism
and the extended family are striking and, at first glance, unexpected. However, the explicit conceptualization of Grebler et al.

(1970) of the extended family as a trigenerational household unit versus the implicit conceptualization of Keefe et al. (1978a, 1978b, 1979) of the modified extended family account for the contrasting findings.

To measure familism, Keefe et al. created an extended family integration scale that included the number of local related households, the frequency of visiting kin, and the extent of mutual aid from relatives. They found that Anglos were massed at the "low integration" end of the scale, whereas Chicanos, particularly the U.S.-born, tended to fall at the upper, "high integration" end of the scale. This correlation between ethnicity and the extended family indicators was quite powerful statistically:

> . . . limiting the sample to those respondents with relatives nearby, the correlations between ethnic group and extended family indicators . . . remain significant when controlling for occupation level, years of education, and years of residence in town. . . . The difference between the two ethnic groups are due mostly to ethnicity rather than class factors. (Keefe et al., 1978a, p. 17)

When the comparative analysis is focused within the Chicano sample, exploring differences by nativity and generations in the United States, it was found that

> . . . the extended family established in the United States by the [Mexican] immigrants increases in size and extent of integration in the second generation and maintains its strength in the third generation. . . . There is no indication of break-down nor emulation of the Anglo American extended family pattern. (Keefe et al., 1978a, p. 19)

In the same study, Keefe et al. (1978a) found that Anglos who do not have relatives in town go to friends for help more often than those Anglos who do have relatives nearby, and that those with kin in town rely on relatives more than those who lack nearby kin. This contrasts with the Mexican-Americans who consult most often with relatives whether or not they have relatives living in town:

> Thus, Mexican Americans consistently rely on relatives most often for emotional support regard-less of their geographic accessibility, while Anglos

turn to friends more often than to relatives when kin
are inaccessible and equally as often when kin are
present. . . . Anglos lack a preference for familial
emotional support. (Keefe et al., 1978a, p. 39)

Similar findings were reported by Wagner and Schaffer
(1980) in their report on two research projects on the social
networks and survival strategies of Mexican-American, Black,
and Anglo female family heads in San Jose, California. Despite
the relatively small samples used in both projects (38 Mexican-
American, Black, and Anglo female family heads in the first and
13 Mexican-American and 13 Black female heads in the second),
the findings from network analysis are significant in their own
right. In the first project, Wagner and Schaffer (1980) studied
the role of the kinship network and found that "the proximity
of the barrios offered social and economic resources, primarily
family members of the Mexican-American women who were not
available to the same extent for the Anglo and Black single
women" (p. 180). In essence, they found ethnic group differences in the socioeconomic vulnerability of the women within
the "female ghetto" census tracts. They report that 60 percent
or more of the Anglos and Blacks had no relatives living in San
Jose, while this was true for only three (10 percent) of the 30
Mexican-American women. Also, the average size of the kinship
network present for the Mexican-Americans was strikingly larger
compared to that of the other women, Chicanos averaged 11 relatives present in the city (some ranged up to 30 or more), whereas
Anglos and Blacks averaged about four.
    In the second project, which focused on a group of female
family heads whose average length of residence in San Jose was
less than three years, Wagner and Schaffer (1980) report that
"for emotional and social support, Mexican Americans reported
turning to relatives, even though they lived in an environment
that provided an unusually high proportion of potential single
parent friends" (p. 186). This was in marked contrast to the
Black mothers, who were highly dependent on the friendship
networks developed within the apartment complex.
    An often neglected function of the Chicano extended family
is in its relation to the process of immigration and migration, such
as to the urban centers of the Midwest. A number of researchers
have pointed out ways in which the Chicano extended family
reduces the level of stress inherent in such a major social transi-
tion (see, for example, Baca Zinn, 1977). Family aid provides
the resources necessary for stabilizing immediate life situations,
as well as possibly serving to counteract the pervasive sense of

inner uncertainty commonly associated with migration. Baca Zinn (1977) in her discussion of Midwest Chicano families concludes:

> . . . it is clear that Chicano migration which has taken place under the auspices of kinship has operated as a primary support mechanism in urban areas. Urban kinship may well be the most crucial processing mechanism in the migration, settlement, and the emerging way of life of Chicanos in the Midwest. (p. 19)

Baca Zinn's (1977) conclusions are supported by a recent report of a comparative study of extended familism among urban Mexican-Americans, Anglos, and Blacks in Kansas City, Missouri (Mindel, 1980). The study is based on data collected in 1974 and involved a sample of 143 Anglos, 160 Blacks, and 152 Mexican-Americans. Mindel's measure of extended familism utilized four indicators: "extensity of presence" as measured by the total number of households of kin living in the area; "intensity of presence" as measured by the extent to which respondents had both nuclear and extended kin in the area; "interaction" as measured by the number of households of kin interacted with at least monthly; and "functionality" as measured by the extent to which respondents were involved in exchange relationships (for example, mutual aid, support, and so forth) with various categories of kin.

Mindel's (1980) findings on extended family integration generally confirm the earlier findings of Keefe et al.: Chicanos exhibit the highest levels of extended familism and Anglos the lowest, with Black respondents falling somewhere in between. This pattern was found for three of the four measures of extended familism, namely, extensity of presence, intensity of presence, and intensity of interaction. With respect to the functionality of interaction, Blacks were found to maintain the most functional relationships with their kin, followed closely by Chicanos, with Anglos trailing far behind. In analyzing the effects of urban migration, Mindel found that

> . . . Anglos who have migrated to this urban area have few kin present, indicating movement away from their relatives. In the case of Mexican Americans, migration appears to be toward areas where kin already are present; the migration process is carried on within the context of the kinship network.

Blacks, as before, appear to fall somewhere in between, not as separate from their relatives as Anglos,
but not as immersed into the kinship network as the
Mexican Americans. (1980, p. 29)

Thus, Chicanos and Anglos have fundamentally different
local kinship structures (Keefe et al., 1979). Anglos tend to
have a very limited local extended family, if they have any at
all. Chicanos, on the other hand, tend to have kin groups comprised of large numbers of local households that are well integrated, and encompass three or more generations.

This apparent "ethnic" difference leads us to ask whether
the difference itself will eventually disappear as Chicanos are
culturally assimilated in the United States. In her study of
acculturation and the extended family among urban Chicanos,
Keefe (1980) points out that as Chicanos become farther and
farther removed generationally from Mexico, they lose significant
awareness of and contact with their cultural heritage, while at
the same time enhancing their awareness of mainstream American
culture. Yet familism, both in terms of values and behaviors,
is at "the core of a culture" and is thus retained and maintained,
while more superficial cultural traits are discarded and forgotten
by succeeding generations (Keefe, 1980). In short, the Chicano
extended family does not necessarily decline with decreasing
cultural awareness and loyalty.

Our review of this small but important body of research
leads us to conclude that the structure and function of Chicano
families are characterized by: a strong, persistent familistic
orientation; a widespread existence of highly integrated extended
kinship systems, even for Chicanos who are three or more generations removed from Mexico; and the consistent preference of
Chicanos for relying on the extended family for support, as the
primary means of coping with emotional stress. In the words
of Temple-Trujillo (1974), in her critical review of past conceptions of the Chicano family,

. . . the strength of the Chicano family seems to be
in the capacity to preserve human relationships and
the satisfaction derived from those interactions . . .
[the extended family] remains a fairly common experience in terms of affective bonds within the Chicano
community. A child growing up within a network of
friends and relatives tends to have many caretakers
and is sensitive to the fact that there exist many
alternative sources of love (p. 18).

Nature of Exchange Relationships among Family Members

We have used a structural definition of the Mexican-American family as "a localized kin group consisting of a number of related households whose members interact together frequently and exchange mutual aid" (Keefe, 1980, p. 89). Past researchers, however, have raised questions about the true extent of mutual aid among Chicano family members, suggesting that exchange among extended family members may be based on values or attitudes about sharing rather than actual exchange (Grebler et al., 1970).

Recent empirical work by Gilbert (1978) sheds new light on both the nature and extent of mutual aid among Chicano family members. For her analysis, Gilbert divides the family into two major categories of kin: primary kin, which includes parents, siblings, and adult children of respondent and spouse; and secondary kin, which includes aunts, uncles, grandparents, first and second cousins, nieces and nephews of the respondent and/or spouse (1978, p. 32). In her study of the kinship relations of 119 second-generation Mexican-Americans living in two Southern California locales, Gilbert (1978) found differences in the geographical distribution of primary versus secondary kin; respondents had greater numbers of primary kin who were geographically more accessible than secondary kin. While this affected the extent of exchange with primary versus secondary kin, other factors seemed also to play a role.

Gilbert collapsed the types of exchange into two general categories: "basic exchange, including financial gifts or loans and the provision of shelter, and personal service exchange, including labor, baby sitting, sickbed care, and personal advice with problems and transportation" (1978, p. 40). She found that "selective recruitment in keeping with the norms of genealogical distance operates in terms of both kinds of exchange and direction of exchange" (p. 41). Basic exchange was carried on almost exclusively with primary kin, while personal service exchange was carried on almost exclusively with secondary kin.

O. Ramírez's (1980) findings were similar with respect to the impact of geographical distribution on extent of exchange. With his sample of 81 Americans of Mexican descent in Detroit, Michigan, he studied two types of aid: non-mental health aid (a category that combines Gilbert's categories of basic and personal service exchange except for personal advice and emotional support) and family mental health aid (a category involving only exchange of emotional support). Using a model that focused on exchange between households among families instead of a primary versus secondary kin model, Ramírez found a high degree of material and emotive interdependency. In essence, he found that the more family one has available, the more types of non-mental health aid one exchanges with them. Likewise, the more family one has available, the greater the number of family members who will be sought out for emotional support. Geographical proximity is thus significantly associated with the level of exchange.

Sena-Rivera's (1979) study suggests another dimension of the nature of exchange relationships among Mexican-American families. He found that among the four extended familias he studied, economic interdependence was "strongest for the most affluent familia and [for] the least affluent, but at the same time, all households of all [four] familias are essentially independent financially" (p. 126). Sena-Rivera further notes that "interdependency in personal services is universal and taken for granted among and within generations, but it follows socioeconomic lines in terms of actual necessity rather than performance as an end itself" (p. 126).

From these few empirical reports, we may conclude that despite variations in the extent of exchange relationships among family systems, real patterns of mutual aid and support are clearly established in the population of Americans of Mexican descent. Geographical distribution of the family, socioeconomic status of the family, and genealogical distance are some of the factors that determine the kind, amount, the target, and direction of the exchange relationship.

Family and Gender Roles

The areas of family and gender roles constitute another major aspect of modern Mexican-American family life that is undergoing considerable reassessment and conceptual reformulation. We are all too familiar with the inadequacies of past research on the Chicano family, such as the lack of solid empirical bases noted above, interpretations based on questionable or racially biased assumptions about Chicano culture. Alvírez and Bean (1976) make the critical point that:

. . . the interpretation of Mexican American family life in terms of monolithic stereo-types implicitly assigns too great a role to the influence of cultural factors in shaping the family patterns of Mexican Americans. It invites the idea that certain patterns

are derivative of beliefs and values passed from
generation to generation rather than functional
adaptations to a difficult environment. (p. 289)

Baca Zinn (1980) noted recently that past research on
changes in Mexican-American families focused on cultural factors
as major determinants while all but ignoring the impact of social
and economic conditions, and consequently, yielded a view of
the process of change as a mere "substitution of modern patterns
for traditional ones" (p. 48). As with families in general, Chicano
family roles are shaped or determined by a wide range of variables, many of which may have little to do with culture per se.
The internal diversity among Chicano family types, as Mirandé
(1977) points out, necessitates consideration of variables such
as "region, recentness of migration to the United States, education, social class, age, and urban-rural locale" (p. 751).
The traditional, stereotypic view of Mexican-American
family and gender roles is commonly characterized by absolute
male dominance and rigid sex/age grading, such that the older
order the younger and the men order the women (Mirandé, 1977).
Miller (1978) provides an excellent summary of the way this
traditional scenario typically unfolds:

Elders command great respect and deference. Sex
roles are rigidly dichotomized with the male conform-
ing to the dominant-agressive archetype, and the
female being the polar opposite—subordinate and
passive. The father is unquestioned patriarch—the
family provider, protector, and judge. His word is
law and demands strict obedience. Presumably, he
is perpetually obsessed with the need to prove his
manhood, often times through excessive drinking,
fighting, and/or extra-marital conquests. The
husband's machismo is strikingly contrasted by the
behavior of his wife. Essentially confined to the
home, she is bound up in all the duties entailed in
being an exemplary wife and mother of a large family.
Her activities beyond the home are limited to frequent
visits with relatives. (pp. 217-18)

While this description may have depicted accurately the
modal Mexican-American family at some point in the past, recent
empirical studies in the areas of male dominance, conjugal decision
making, and the role of the woman in the family suggest that
Chicano families have undergone and are currently undergoing

substantial changes along these dimensions. Furthermore, as stated earlier, these changes cannot be attributed simplistically to a supposedly uniform process of acculturation. As the studies reviewed below indicate, we can no longer accept as viable the framework which holds that as Chicano families move generationally through time, they become acculturated and reach an end point as a "modern American family" and thus cease to be "ethnic." Chicano families can be modern and ethnic at the same time (Baca Zinn, 1980). Some of the characteristics of Chicano family and gender roles to be discussed are not necessarily recent changes as such, but are actually characteristics that may have been normative for quite some time but may not have been empirically observed and reported to date. These characteristics seem novel largely as the result of the reexamination and reformulation by Chicano scholars of earlier data employing new and broader frameworks that do not inherently presume pathology and deficiency in the Mexican-American family and by the increasing use of systematic empirical data rather than descriptive and nonrepresentative data.

Male Dominance in Conjugal Decision Making

Central to the traditional depiction of Chicano family roles is the issue of patriarchal structure, the absolute dominance of the male in the family. The emphasis on this characteristic has persisted despite an increasing amount of evidence to the contrary. A number of researchers have suggested that the patterns of absolute male dominance in conjugal decision making have never been the behavioral norm among Mexicans either in the United States or Mexico (Cromwell & Ruiz, 1979; Hawkes & Taylor, 1975; Grebler et al., 1970). The evidence presented by these researchers generally suggests the presence of a more egalitarian structure and process than is commonly supposed for Mexican and Chicano families.

Cromwell and Ruiz (1979) conducted an intensive analysis or reanalysis of four major studies on marital decision making within Mexican and Chicano families. The studies analyzed by Cromwell and Ruiz (1979) consisted of four separate, cross-national data sets on conjugal decision making based on samples of Mexican wives and husbands (Cromwell, Corrales, & Torsiello, 1973; de Lenero, 1969), Chicano wives (Hawkes & Taylor, 1975), and Chicano wives and husbands (Cromwell & Cromwell, 1978).[2] Their review of these four studies did not support the notion of male dominance in marital decision making. They concluded, "basically, the studies suggest that while wives make the fewest unilateral decisions and husbands make more, joint decisions are by far the most common in these samples of Mexican, Chicano, and Anglo working-class people" (Cromwell & Ruiz, 1979, p. 370).

Other recent studies by Ybarra-Soriano (1977) and Baca Zinn (1980) also confirm the tendency of joint decision making behavior to coexist with the entrenched patriarchal ideology; but more importantly, these studies provide us with new insights into factors that may play a more determinant role. Ybarra-Soriano (1977) conducted intensive interviews focusing on conjugal role relationships with 100 Chicano married couples broadly representative of the Chicano population in Fresno, California. Her results indicated that the Chicano families showed a wide range of conjugal role patterns, from a patriarchal to an egalitarian structure, but the majority of Chicano married couples shared decision making. In her analysis of the variables that might affect the type of conjugal role structure, Ybarra-Soriano found no statistically significant correlations between level of acculturation, educational attainment, or income level and the type of conjugal role relationship. However, she did find that wives' employment outside the home had a strong impact on conjugal role structure: If the wife worked outside the home, there was a greater likelihood that she would have a greater role in decision making and, thus, such couples would have a more joint conjugal role structure than couples in which the wife was not employed.

In recent study, Baca Zinn (1980) examined the effect of wives' employment outside the home and level of education on conjugal interaction. The study, which was conducted in an urban New Mexico setting over a ten-month period in 1975, involved intensive interviewing and observation of eight Mexican-American families, four with employed wives and four with nonemployed wives. Middle-class and working-class families were equally represented. Also, families were essentially at the same stage of the family life cycle: all had teenage children and some grade school children and/or adult children. It is also important to note that all the employed wives had or were in the process of completing a four-year college degree.

In general, Baca Zinn's findings indicate that there were differences in family power between families with employed and nonemployed wives: "In all families where women were not employed, tasks and decision making were typically sex-segregated. However, in all families with employed wives, tasks and decision-making were shared" (1980, p. 51). Interestingly, despite the power differential between employed and nonemployed wives, the ideology of patriarchy was strongly asserted in all eight families. She comments that "finding that families could be patriarchal in ideology but not in practice points to the need to distinguish between traditional values and actual behavior" (1980, p. 52).

Baca Zinn's (1980) findings regarding the level of ethnicity of the families studied are both remarkable and important for their theoretical implications. All of the families in the study shared similarities in their use of the Spanish language, their preference for Mexican and Spanish food, and their choice of Spanish or Mexican music. Clearly, such a finding, considered in conjunction with Ybarra-Soriano's (1977) study, provides a firm basis for questioning the assumption that shifts away from traditional conjugal roles in Mexican-American families are a result of acculturation and a corresponding decrease in the level of ethnicity.

While further research is needed to determine the extent to which "differences in conjugal relationships result from cultural values surrounding roles and to what extent they result from specific socioeconomic conditions including educational and occupational statuses of husbands and wives" (Baca Zinn, 1980, p. 59), the findings we have presented here indicate that the single variable of the wife's employment outside the home has a substantial impact on conjugal roles. An important question at this juncture is how widespread such an impact might be among the population of Americans of Mexican descent, with its steadily accelerating rate of female participation in the labor force.

As indicated earlier, the rate of Chicana participation in the paid labor force has increased dramatically over the past decade from below 30 percent in 1970 to over 45 percent at present. The combined effects of the pace of the change over the past decade and the actual level of present labor force participation must be viewed as a key variable affecting Chicano family life, both now and in the future. Also as Mirandé and Enríquez (1979) point out, these data effectively counter the myth of the Chicana as primarily a traditional homemaker.

Machismo

Just as current research is beginning to dispel many myths about the role of women in Mexican-American families, we are also beginning to get a clearer, more accurate view of the roles of Mexican-American men, as husbands and fathers. Traditionally, Chicano males have been associated with the concept of "machismo." Indeed, the use of the Spanish word as the label for this concept implies that this is primarily a Mexican or Latin American phenomenon. This notion stresses absolute patriarchy, exaggerated masculinity, and sexual virility—particularly in the extramarital sphere. There is a growing body of evidence that suggests that this is a "grossly exaggerated misrepresentation" and "men that fit this description, and they do exist among Mexican Americans just as they do in all ethnic groups, are the exception rather than the norm" (Valdez, 1980, p. 4). For example, in Ybarra-Soriano's (1977) study, the majority of respondents reacted negatively to the type of behavior described by the traditional definition of machismo. Ybarra-Soriano concluded from this that "the concept of machismo, as it has been defined in social science literature, should not be regarded as an integral part of Chicano culture and, as such, should not be seen as the basis for male-female roles within the family" (1977, p. 86).

It is generally recognized that machismo as an exaggerated version of masculinity is cross-cultural and constitutes an aberration or a form of individual deviancy and consequently is rarely normative in any cultural group. The adoption of egalitarian conjugal behavior among a growing number of Chicano couples is quite at odds with the concept of machismo as traditionally defined. Perhaps what is needed is a reformulation or redefinition of the concept that would describe more accurately, and indeed, less pejoratively, the Mexican-American male and his role in the family. R. Ramírez (1979) suggests that such a definition might include "such positive cultural characteristics as respect, honesty, loyalty, fairness, responsibility, and trustworthiness" (pp. 61-62). Similarly Alvírez and Bean (1976) suggest that the concept of machismo encompasses manliness in a broader sense than mere sexual prowess and includes "the elements of courage, honor, and respect for others as well as the notion of providing fully for one's family and maintaining close ties with the extended family" (p. 278).

Recent research on the role of the father in the Chicano family also serves to effectively counter the negative, derogatory view of the Mexican-American male. Lúzod (1978), for example, studied the division of household labor within the home as well as child nurturing tasks within the home. His sample consisted of 37 female and 26 male respondents of Mexican ancestry from Detroit, Michigan. Among his findings was that housework within the Chicano family is a group effort, with children of both sexes helping one another. Results of normative value statements

indicated that mothers and fathers were in complete agreement
that childrearing is as important to men as it is to women. Luzód
points out that:

> When it comes to the father's reported involvement
> in child nurturing tasks, it is clear that this domain
> is not solely the responsibility of the mother. Fathers
> as well as mothers strongly stress the importance of
> education, being involved in the children's activities,
> and discussing career goals. Fathers, however,
> report more encouragement for children to do things
> for himself/herself. (1978, pp. 8-9)

The results point again to the notion of a more democratic,
egalitarian approach to family roles among Chicanos, which
necessitates not only a reconsideration of the role of women in
the Chicano family, but also the role of men. According to Grebler
et al. (1970),

> . . . though the Mexican American man may still
> refuse to wash dishes, in the more important aspects
> of the husband-wife and father-child relationship
> he is willing to admit that he has ceded control;
> at the same time he has assumed some of the respon-
> sibilities that were traditionally "feminine." (p. 363)

SUMMARY AND CONCLUSION

Empirical research indicates that Chicanos and Anglos have
substantially different local kinship structures. Chicanos have
local kin in more households and the families in these households
are more fully integrated and are more likely to encompass several
generations. Generally familistic values and behaviors seem to
resist Chicano cultural and structural assimilation. The evidence
for the Chicano extended family as socially and emotionally supportive is persuasive and Chicanos are found to actually prefer
and to receive substantial familial support over alternative sources
of support. Though not conclusively demonstrated, familial
support may also lessen the vulnerability of Chicano family members, for example, in relation to the stress of immigration and
migration.

Although traditional patriarchy as the predominant norm
for Chicano families is being gradually displaced by egalitarianism, such a shift cannot be reductionistically attributed to

acculturation. Instead, wives' educational attainment and employment outside the home are stronger determinants of egalitarian decision making. Further, changes in conjugal role structure do not require a decline in level of ethnicity, i.e., Chicano families can be modern and ethnic at the same time (Baca Zinn, 1980). Most of the exaggerated masculinity behaviors generally included within the rubric of machismo are pancultural but constitute forms of individual deviancy and are rarely normative in any culture. Further empirical study should focus on the Chicano male in his roles as father and husband, and will hopefully produce new conceptualizations that are neither pejorative nor pathological in their views of Chicanos.

Current research interest on Chicano family life has originated primarily in response to the dearth of adequate empirical data. Prior to 1970, Chicano family literature was sparse and empirically deficient. It argued that the family was old-fashioned, structurally rigid, male-dominated, unresponsive to the demands of contemporary industrial society, and detrimental to individual mobility and coping ability. In the past decade a new body of literature argued that the Chicano family is a tenacious and adaptable instrument for Chicanos confronting an often hostile society and environment. The empirical base for these more recent views, although neither extensive nor conclusive, has not been adequately reviewed. We have attempted this integrative review and have extracted some of the more significant findings on Chicano family life. These findings portray a distinctive institution that has been and continues to be dynamic, creative, and supportive.

NOTES

1. Although there is a considerable body of secondary literature based on demographic statistics about Chicanos and Chicano families, this portrait is based exclusively on primary data from the following U.S. Bureau of the Census documents: 1970 Census of Population, Persons of Spanish Origin PC(2)-1C, Family Composition, PC(2)-4A; Current Population Reports, Fertility of American Women: June 1977 (P-20, No. 235), Marital Status and Living Arrangements: March, 1979 (P-20, No. 349), Persons of Spanish Origin in the United States: March 1977 (P-20, No. 329), and Persons of Spanish Origin in the United States: March 1978 (P-20, No. 339); and A Statistical Portrait of Women in the United States: 1978 (P-23, No. 100).

2. The studies selected by Cromwell and Ruiz (1979) for reexamination were: Cromwell, R. E., Corrales, R. G., &

Torsiello, P. M., Normative patterns of marital decision making
power and influence in Mexico and the United States: A partial
test of resource and ideology theory, Journal of Comparative
Family Studies, 1973, 4, 177-96; Cromwell, V. L., & Cromwell,
R. E., Perceived dominance in decision making and conflict
resolution among Anglo, Black and Chicano couples, Journal of
Marriage and the Family, 1978, 40, 749-59; de Lenero, D. C. E.,
Hacia Donde Va La Mujer Mexicana? Mexico City: Instituto Mexicano de Estudios Sociales, 1969; Hawkes, G. R., & Taylor, M.,
Power structure in Mexican and Mexican-American farm labor
families, Journal of Marriage and the Family, 1975, 37, 807-11.

REFERENCES

Alvírez, D., & Bean, F. D. The Mexican American family. In
C. H. Mindel & R. W. Habenstein (Eds.), Ethnic families in
America. New York: Elsevier, 1976, pp. 271-92.

Árce, C. H. Dimensions of familism and familial identification.
Paper presented at the C.O.S.S.M.H.O. Conference on the
Hispanic family, Houston, Tex., October 1978.

Baca Zinn, M. Urban kinship and midwest Chicano families:
Review and reformulation. Paper prepared for presentation
at the annual meeting of the Western Social Science Association,
Denver, Colo., April 23, 1977.

Baca Zinn, M. Employment and education of Mexican-American
women: The interplay of modernity and ethnicity in eight
families. Harvard Educational Review, 1980, 50, No. 1, 47-62.

Bennett, J. W., & Despres, L. A. Kinship and instrumental
activities: A theoretical inquiry. American Anthropologist,
1960, 62, 254-67.

Cromwell, R., & Ruiz, R. A. The myth of macho dominance in
decision making within Mexican and Chicano families. Hispanic
Journal of Behavioral Sciences, December 1979, 1, No. 4,
355-73.

Gilbert, M. J. Extended family integration among second genera-
tion Mexican Americans. In J. M. Casas & S. E. Keefe (Eds.),
Family and mental health in the Mexican American community.
Los Angeles: Spanish Speaking Mental Health Research Center,
UCLA, Monograph No. 7, 1978, pp. 25-48.

Grebler, L., Moore, J. W., & Guzmán, R. C. The Mexican American people: The nation's second largest minority. New York: The Free Press, 1970.

Hawkes, G. R., & Taylor, M. Power structure in Mexican and Mexican-American farm labor families. Journal of Marriage and the Family, 1975, 37, 807-11.

Keefe, S. E. Acculturation and the extended family among urban Mexican Americans. In A. M. Padilla (Ed.), Acculturation: Theory, models, and some new findings. Boulder: Westview Press, 1980, pp. 85-110.

Keefe, S. E., Padilla, A. M., & Carlos, M. L. Emotional support systems in two cultures: A comparison of Mexican Americans and Anglo Americans. Los Angeles: Spanish Speaking Mental Health Research Center, UCLA, 1978, Occasional Paper No. 7. (a)

Keefe, S. E., Padilla, A. M., & Carlos, M. L. The Mexican American extended family as an emotional support system. In J. M. Casas & S. E. Keefe (Eds.), Family and mental health in the Mexican American community. Los Angeles: Spanish Speaking Mental Health Research Center, UCLA, 1978, Monograph No. 7, pp. 49-67. (b)

Keefe, S. E., Padilla, A. M., & Carlos, M. L. The Mexican-American extended family as an emotional support system. Human Organization, Summer 1979, 38, No. 2, 144-52.

Litwak, E. Occupational mobility and extended family cohesion. American Sociological Review, February 1960, 25, 9-21. (a)

Litwak, E. Geographic mobility and extended family cohesion. American Sociological Review, June 1960, 25, 385-94. (b)

Litwak, E. Extended kin relations in an industrial democratic society. In Ethel Shanas & Gordon F. Streib (Eds.), Social structure and the family: Generational relations. Englewood Cliffs: Prentice-Hall, 1965, pp. 290-323.

Luzód, J. A. The role of the father in la familia Chicana. Paper presented at the C.O.S.S.M.H.O. Conference on the Hispanic Family, Houston, Tex., October 1978.

Miller, M. V. Variations in Mexican American family life: A review synthesis of empirical research. Aztlan: International Journal of Chicano Studies Research, 1978, 9, 209-31.

Mindel, C. H. Extended familism among urban Mexican Americans, Anglos and Blacks. Hispanic Journal of Behavioral Sciences, March 1980, 2, No. 1, 21-34.

Mirandé, A. The Chicano family; A reanalysis of conflicting views. Journal of Marriage and the Family, November 1977, 747-56.

Mirandé, A., & Enríquez, E. La Chicana: The Mexican American woman. Chicago: The University of Chicago Press, 1979.

Ramírez, O. Extended family phenomena and mental health among urban Mexican Americans. Latino Institute, Monograph No. 3, Reston, Virginia: November 1980.

Ramírez, R. Machismo: A bridge rather than a barrier to family and marital counseling. In P. P. Martin (Ed.), La frontera perspective: Providing mental health services to Mexican Americans. Tucson: La Frontera Center, 1979, pp. 61-62.

Sena, J. R. The survival of the Mexican extended family in the United States: Evidence from a Southern California town. Ph.D. dissertation, University of California, Los Angeles, 1973. University Microfilms No. 73-18, 651.

Sena-Rivera, J. Casa and Familia: An alternative model of the traditional Chicano extended family—A report on exploratory investigation. Paper read at the Annual Meeting of the American Sociological Association, New York, August 1976.

Sena-Rivera, J. La familia Chicana as a mental health resource: A trigenerational study of four Mexican descent extended families in the Michigan-Indiana-Illinois region. Advance report, Department of Sociology and Anthropology, University of Notre Dame, Notre Dame, Ind., 1977.

Sena-Rivera, J. Extended kinship in the United States: Competing models and the case of la familia Chicana. Journal of Marriage and the Family, February 1979, 121-29.

Temple-Trujillo, R. E. Conceptions of the Chicano family. Smith College Studies in Social Work, 1974, 45, No. 7.

Valdez, R. The Mexican American male: A brief review of the literature. Newsletter of the Mental Health Research Project, I.D.R.A., San Antonio, Winter 1980, 4-5.

Wagner, R. M., & Schaffer, D. M. Social networks and survival strategies: An exploratory study of Mexican American, Black, and Anglo female family heads in San Jose, California. In M. B. Melville (Ed.), Twice a minority: Mexican American women. St. Louis: C. V. Mosby, 1980, pp. 173-90.

Ybarra-Soriano, L. Conjugal role relationships in the Chicano family. Unpublished Ph.D. dissertation, University of California at Berkeley, 1977.

2

THE HISPANIC ELDERLY:
A REVIEW OF HEALTH, SOCIAL,
AND PSYCHOLOGICAL FACTORS

Frank Cota-Robles Newton

The field of Hispanic gerontology began in earnest in the early 1970s. Thus, with the advent of a new decade, it seems a propitious moment to assess the findings of the past ten years with an eye toward the proper direction of research and service delivery in the next ten.

As a starting point, the most basic observation that can be made is that the 1970s were primarily a time for the training of the first, small cadre of Hispanic gerontology professionals. One consequence of this is that a sizable number of research reports generated during the decade were master's theses and doctoral dissertations.[1] Concomitantly, these investigations were descriptive studies based on surveys with small sample sizes, reflecting the youth of the researchers and their limited access to research money and related resources.

Second, an understandable and seemingly pervasive feeling was that the subject of Hispanic elderly was a great unknown. This, too, prompted a spate of exploratory, descriptive studies. The result was a number of worthwhile reports, filled with demographic data and revealing insights into the customs, characteristics, and needs of Hispanic elderly. However, being exploratory and nonexperimental, these studies were not readily generalizable nor theoretically well-grounded; consequently, their data were open to a variety of contradictory interpretations.[2]

In light of these circumstances, it is very clear that in this new decade of Hispanic gerontology we must build upon the learning experiences and exploratory ventures of the past. Specifically, this means that experimental research as well as longitudinal and ethnographic studies must replace the all too prevalent surveys. More programmatic research is necessary, as opposed to the many past studies that were formulated in isolation from each other. Most importantly, there must be research that leads to new, culturally appropriate theoretical models, especially models that recognize the complex interaction of a multiplicity of variables.

To promote these necessary developments in the field, the following discussion will organize, review, and summarize the available literature on Hispanic elderly. Moreover, to provide an overview that is as comprehensive as possible, the findings will be arranged according to the three most global factors in the social sciences: health, social, and psychological factors.

HEALTH FACTOR

General Health Status

In the early and mid-1970s there were several claims in the literature that poor health was a common and severe problem among Hispanic more than nonminority elderly in the United States (Hill, 1975; Torres-Gil, 1978; White House, 1971). It is most unfortunate that now, half a dozen years later, there are still no firm, empirical data to substantiate these claims, for as yet there have been no major studies on the incidence and preva- lence of specific ailments and disabilities among Hispanic elderly. Nevertheless, those early claims are much more compelling at present because there have been a number of studies measuring Hispanic elders' self-perceived state of health. All of these studies document that poor health is one of the most serious and prevalent problems in this population. For example, two surveys conducted in Texas (Blau, 1978; Steglich, Cartwright, & Crouch, 1968) report that health was a high-priority need among Mexican-American elderly. In Valle and Mendoza's (1978) San Diego, California, survey, 36 percent of their elderly Mexican- American sample rated poor health as their major problem, with 39 percent rating their own health as "poor" or "very poor." Similarly, an East Los Angeles study (Castro, Dehmer, Edmond, Hernández, Larios, Ramos, Torres, & Wincowski, 1978) found that poor health was the major complaint of elderly Mexican- Americans, with the majority of respondents rating their health as "poor" or no better than "fair." Finally, a large-scale study in Los Angeles conducted by the University of Southern California Andrus Gerontology Center produced a number of findings that document the severity of health problems among elderly Mexican- Americans: first, 48 percent listed health as their major problem in life (Ragan & Simonin, 1977); second, compared to a mere 4 percent of the Anglo elderly respondents, 28 percent of the aged Mexican-Americans rated their health as "poor" or "very poor" (Cooper, Simonin, & Newquist, 1978); third, Mexican-American elderly reported more health-related difficulties in performing daily tasks, including holding a regular job, than Anglo elderly (Newquist, Berger, Kahn, Martínez, & Burton, 1979); and fourth, Mexican-American elderly were more likely than Anglo elderly to cite "poor health" as a reason for retirement, with 34 percent of the Mexican-American respondents who were age 45 to 49 already reporting that they suffered health problems that hampered them from holding a regular job (Newquist et al., 1979).

Very clearly, the mounting evidence strongly indicates that illnesses and disabilities are a more pronounced and prevalent problem for Mexican-American than nonminority elderly and, moreover, that they are experiencing these problems at a much younger age. In light of such evidence, more research as well as more health services for these elders is definitely needed. Nevertheless, it must be emphasized that future studies must be more carefully focused and specific about types of health problems because the global measure of self-rated health in no way effectively discriminates between ailments that vary by chronicity or the degree of threat to life (for example, arthritis versus cancer; hearing impairment versus high blood pressure). Certainly more health services are imperative, but they cannot be properly planned and channeled until precise incidence and prevalence data are available.

Health-related Variables

A better understanding of elderly Hispanics' health problems can only be obtained by considering the context within which these problems develop and are experienced. Specifically, this refers to several key variables that either cause or complicate poor health within this population or subsets of the population.

Work History

In the East Los Angeles study previously cited (Castro et al., 1978), it was found that two-thirds of the elderly Mexican-American male respondents had spent most of their lives in blue-collar or unskilled jobs, and 96 percent of the female respondents had held either domestic or unskilled jobs. These findings correspond to census data showing that on the whole, Chicanos occupy the lowest occupational levels, with the preponderant majority in blue-collar, service, or farm jobs (U.S. Census, 1976).

The health-related significance of this is that such jobs tend to be physically exhausting and debilitating. It is not surprising, therefore, to learn from the Andrus Gerontology Study that compared to 24 percent of Anglo male respondents, 64 percent of the Mexican-American males had to retire because of physical disabilities (Ragan and Simonin, 1977). Moreover, these disabilities, and the consequent retirement, occur at an earlier age for Mexican-Americans (Newquist et al., 1979). The implication is that a large number of Mexican-Americans are entering old age suffering from physical disabilities and other forms of poor health.

Sex Differences

There are two studies that report sex differences in the health status of Mexican-American elderly. First, a New Mexico study by Korte (1978) found that poor health may be more common among men than women in this population, especially in urban areas. Specifically, Korte's rural respondents generally tended to rate their health as at least "fair," while the urban respondents tended to rate their health as "poor." Moreover, the majority of the urban females rated their health as at least "fair" while 65 percent of the urban males rated their health as "poor" or "very poor." In contrast to these findings, a statewide telephone survey of elderly persons in Texas (Blau, 1978) found that the health of Mexican-American women was somewhat worse than the men's, although the sex difference was not statistically significant.

There is no clear-cut explanation for the different results obtained by these two studies because the authors do not provide sufficient information. But it can be conjectured that Korte's findings make sense in terms of Clark's (1971) conclusion that city life is much more damaging than rural life to the health of elderly persons. There is support, as well, from the Los Angeles study previously mentioned, which found that many Mexican-American males must retire from work because of poor health. On the other hand, there is support for Blau's finding in her own observation that elderly Mexican-American women have poorer health than men because "they have devoted their entire adult lives to bearing and rearing many children" (1978, p. 14). The conclusion that must necessarily be drawn from these two studies is that future research must examine the health-related life history differences of Hispanic men and women. Moreover, it is clear from this case that the global measure of self-rated health is inadequate to get an accurate picture of elderly Hispanics' health problems. What is called for, again, is specific information on the types of ailments suffered by men and women in this population in addition to rural-urban differences in the health of elderly Hispanics.

Poverty

There have been numerous studies documenting that elderly Hispanics are "the poorest of the poor," being significantly poorer than nonminority elderly.[3] One ramification of this is that poor nutrition may be a serious problem. For example, by inference, it seems significant that LeBovit's (1965) study reports that the poorest diets are found among the oldest and poorest homemakers. Furthermore, Garcia-Mohr (1979) asserts that because of their very small, fixed incomes and their illnesses which limit their mobility to shop, Mexican-American elderly may be at a higher risk of malnutrition than other elders.

A second problem is that poverty limits elderly Mexican-Americans' access to medical resources. Several studies have found that because of their unskilled or migrant job histories, Mexican-American elders are significantly less likely to receive Social Security; and as a direct consequence, they are less likely to receive Medicare benefits (Santos, in press). Moreover, according to the Andrus Gerontology study, low-income, minority elderly are less likely to have health insurance, with 4 percent of the Mexican-American elders interviewed having no health insurance at all (Newquist et al., 1979). Although they are more at risk of health problems, Mexican-American elderly are also more at risk of encountering financial barriers to health care.

An even more insidious problem is that when low-income, minority elderly do have health insurance, it is most likely that they rely primarily or exclusively on government health insurance. The difficulty with this is that such insurance is not geared to the needs of the elderly. Besides having numerous restrictions, gaps, and other limitations, government health plans are basically designed for acute or episodic illnesses, not the chronic health problems suffered by the elderly. Therefore, in light of the fact that placement in a long-term care facility may often be necessary to receive government health coverage for chronic, although relatively minor health problems, those elderly who must rely exclusively on government health insurance are especially at risk of institutionalization (Newquist et al., 1979).

SOCIAL FACTOR

Natural Support Systems

Although innumerable studies of Chicano culture have documented the paramount social and psychological importance of la familia (the family), there is a major controversy in the Hispanic gerontology literature concerning the extent to which the family has remained tightly integrated and supportive of the elderly. At the heart of the controversy is modernization theory, which postulates that as urbanization and industrialization increase so do social and geographic mobility; and concomitantly, there occurs dissipation and disorganization of family networks.[4]

On one side of the argument are several authors who contend that the Hispanic family system is breaking down (Maldonado, 1975; Atencio, 1976; Galarza, in press). Basically, their argument is that Mexican-Americans' recent mass exodus from rural to urban life, compounded by the increased education, income, and acculturation of the new generation, have created a rift in the traditional Mexican values of family unity and support for elders.

Contraposed to this argument is the position that the Mexican-American family is, indeed, changing but it is not breaking down. A number of studies, for example, have documented that Mexican-American elderly are much more likely to be living independently than in another person's home (Acosta, 1975; Castro et al., 1978; J. B. Cuéllar, 1978; Estrada, 1977; Valle & Mendoza, 1978). But the important point is that they are not living entirely alone but, instead, with a spouse, children or grandchildren, and/or within the same neighborhood as their children (Carp, 1969; Keefe, Padilla, & Carlos, 1979; Sotomayor, 1973). What this body of evidence indicates is that the traditional, essentially rural pattern of multigeneration households is being replaced in urban settings with, what Litwak (1965) terms, "modified extended families." Thus, Hispanic elderly in cities seem to prefer their independence, while maintaining close, regular contact with their relatives.

Complementing this latter position is an increasingly significant line of inquiry on natural support systems beyond the immediate family (Mendoza, 1979a, 1979b; Valle & Martínez, in press; Valle & Mendoza, 1978). The point of these studies is that besides la familia, Hispanic culture has other indigenous, helping systems that can bolster support for needy elderly. One type, termed "link person networks" by Valle and Martínez (in press), consists of friends or neighbors who are acknowl-

edged in the community as willing and reliable servidoras
(helpers) or consejeras (counselors) for emotional support,
information brokerage, or referral to formal, social service
agencies. A second type of natural support is "aggregate
group networks," including church groups, senior citizen clubs,
sociedades de aseguranza (insurance cooperatives), and other
community groups (J. B. Cuéllar, 1977, 1978). As Mendoza
(1979a) and Valle and Martínez (in press) explain, what is special
about these helping networks is that they are culturally sanctioned and therefore compatible with the distinctive needs and
expectations of Hispanic elders. Moreover, they are vitally
important for mitigating scarce support resources for the elderly,
either by helping an isolated elder when family support does,
in fact, break down or else by providing support where no public
or private social services are available in the community.

To summarize, at present there is no resolution to the
controversy about the extent of family support available to Hispanic elders. What is clear is that modernization has definitely
caused stresses and changes in Hispanic family life, but still
the family as well as the community have been resilient—modifying
to meet new demands, but not breaking down entirely. Future
research, therefore, should not promote the two extremes of the
controversy but, instead, identify with precision those circumstances and variables that foster or undermine the family support
of Hispanic elders.

Formal Support Systems

The steadily mounting evidence in the Hispanic gerontology
literature documents a large number of barriers to the utilization
of health, mental health, and social service providers, with a
clear distinction between Hispanic elders' preference for family
and community support and their reluctance to utilize formal
services. Despite Clark's (1971) observation that inner city
barrios (Hispanic enclaves) are commonly characterized by
poverty, substandard housing, and crime, the work of other
researchers reveals that the barrio is a valuable "cultural coping
mechanism" (J. B. Cuéllar, 1978). In particular, the barrio is
a place where the traditional culture is preserved; it provides
a sense of community, a sense of belonging and cohesion, it is
a secure place where recent immigrants can gradually adapt;
and it is a place where the elder can remain close to children
and grandchildren (Carp, 1969; Manuel & Bengston, 1976; Ragan,
1978; Sotomayor, 1972, 1973; Torres-Gíl, Newquist, & Simonin,

1978). Furthermore, the barrio serves as a psychologically beneficial buffer against the discrimination that many Hispanic elderly
have suffered (Kasschau, 1977; Moore, 1971; Torres-Gíl &
Becerra, 1977).

When one contrasts these positive qualities of the barrio
with the many barriers to formal services, it is not surprising
to find that underutilization of services by Hispanic elderly is
common. For example, an East Los Angeles study found that
whereas over 90 percent of the Mexican American elderly respondents relied on local physicians, less than half utilized the county
hospital, less than one-third used local health or welfare agencies,
and only 1 percent utilized mental health clinics (Castro et al.,
1978). Similarly, one Texas study found that of 390 elderly
surveyed, including Mexican-Americans, only 23 percent used
local medical facilities; they complained that the services only
catered to the young; there were long waits at clinics; and,
especially, the Mexican-American elderly could not understand
the Anglo-American doctors (Reich, Stegman, & Stegman, 1966).

In an effort to clarify this issue of barriers to service
utilization, Salcido (1979a) offers a three-part typology: person
barriers, including lack of education, lack of knowledge about
services, negative attitudes about institutions, and poor health
which isolates the person; environmental barriers, including
geographic isolation, lack of transportation, and lack of services
in the community; and institutional barriers, including restrictive
eligibility requirements, insensitivity by staff to Mexican-American
culture, and language problems. To these critical institutional
barriers can be added six others, identified by the Andrus
Gerontology Study as particularly inhibiting for low-income
minority elderly: physicians refusing to accept Medicaid patients;
government failure to enforce laws prohibiting discrimination
against minority patients by hospitals; regional disparities in
Medicaid eligibility and benefits; restrictive conditions attached
to reimbursement of home health care services; limitations in
services reimbursable under Medicaid or Medicare; and physician
refusal to provide services on assignment through the Medicare
program (Newquist et al., 1979). Finally, a special problem for
a large number of Mexican-American elderly is their illegal alien
status, which effectively prevents their utilization of most public
services (Salcido, 1979b, 1980).

In view of these numerous, often overwhelming, barriers
to service utilization that have already been identified by social
scientists, it does not seem that more research is required.
Instead, since we know what the problems are, what is needed
is legislative intervention as well as greater sensitivity on the

part of service providers. Recognizing this, Salcido (1979a) calls on health service workers to practice "health advocacy" on behalf of Mexican-American elderly including: recognizing and fighting for consumers' rights; ensuring that hospital and clinic environments are conducive to patient well-being, including appropriateness for Mexican-American values and customs; and maintaining regular contact between the agency and the Mexican-American community (J. B. Cuéllar, 1979). Second, more active outreach efforts are required of service providers. Carp's (1970) study, for example, discovered that Mexican-American elderly rely primarily upon relatives for information about community services; therefore, providers must establish linkages with community residents to advertise their services. Similarly, a recent study in Miami among Cuban elders found that advertisements in the Spanish-speaking mass media, especially television, were very effective for increasing utilization at a mental health clinic (Szapocznik, Lasaga, Perry, & Solomon, 1979). Finally, Mendoza (1979a) and Valle & Martínez (in press) have strongly advocated in legislative hearings that human services should and could be more accessible to Hispanic elders by making those services more culturally relevant. This can easily be accomplished, they explain, by using the barrio's natural helping network (that is, the servidora system) as a parallel and supportive system working alongside formal agencies. Clearly such a policy is worthwhile, being cost-effective while also reducing barriers to utilization by promoting culturally sensitive and appropriate services.

PSYCHOLOGICAL FACTOR

Perceptions of Aging

The few studies examining the issue of subjective age among elderly Hispanics concur that Mexican-Americans perceive an early onset to old age (Steglich, Cartwright, & Crouch, 1968). Clark and Anderson (1967) report a majority of Mexican-Americans sampled in San Francisco indicated old age begins as early as age 45. In East Los Angeles, Mexican-Americans were found to consider old age as beginning at age 50 (Bengston, Cuéllar, & Ragan, 1977). In the same study, 30 percent of the Mexican-American respondents considered themselves "old" by age 57, whereas 30 percent of the Anglos not until age 70 (Bengston, 1977). Crouch's (1972) Texas study of Mexican-Americans revealed that the majority believed old age to start below age 60, with 45 percent specifying ages 50 to 55 as the period when old age begins. In the same vein, research indicates that Mexican-Americans who are age 45 or more give a much lower longevity estimate for themselves than do Anglos or Blacks (Reynolds & Kalish, 1974).

Clark and Anderson (1967) theorize that the perception of onset of old age consists of an interaction between actual age and some symbolic event. For Mexican-Americans the single most significant "symbolic event" appears to be poor health, especially poor health that prohibits continued employment. The Andrus Gerontology Study found that among Mexican-Americans aged 65 or more, the majority in poor health considered themselves "old," while those in good health more often described themselves as "middle aged" or even "young" (Cooper, Simonin, & Newquist, 1978). Regarding more precise criteria of old age, Crouch (1972) lists several statements by elderly Mexican-Americans: "poor health," "when one needs help," "when one feels useless," and "when one can no longer work." Valle and Mendoza (1978) also found that for Mexican-Americans "feeling old" is a function of poor physical health as well as an inability to continue working.

To summarize, all the available data agree that Mexican-Americans consider themselves old at a relatively young age (usually before age 60) and also estimate for themselves a fairly short life span because of poor health and years of hard physical labor. Moreover, their poor health and inability to work seem to impact negatively on their adjustment to old age, suggested by their expressions of feeling "helpless" and useless." Thus, the implication is that Mexican-American elderly, at least those who are in poor health, should be expected to have very negative perceptions about growing old.[5]

Morale & Mental Health

In accord with the implications of the "perceptions of aging" data just cited are several studies which suggest that low morale, dissatisfaction with life, and mental health problems may be common among Hispanic elderly. A Houston study, for example, of elderly Anglos, Blacks, and Mexican-Americans found that even though "joy" decreased with age for all three ethnic groups, the Mexican-American elderly reported more depression and lower levels of positive affect, happiness, and contentment than young Mexican-Americans (Gaitz & Scott, 1974; Scott & Gaitz, 1975). Similarly, a Los Angeles study found that Mexican-Americans, especially those over age 65, had much lower "tranquility" scores than Anglos or Blacks; and while tranquility tended to increase with age for Anglos, it decreased with age among Mexican-Americans (Dowd & Bengston, 1974).

Optimism, as another facet of morale, was measured in terms of "positive potential for older persons" by the Andrus Gerontology Study, and it was discovered that compared to Anglos and Blacks, Mexican-Americans had the least positive perceptions of old age (Bengston, 1977; Morgan & Bengston, 1976). Interviewing just the females in the Andrus sample, Ragan (1978) learned that the Mexican-American women were the "unhappiest" and most pessimistic, with only 48 percent of the Mexican-American women, compared to 66 percent of the Black women, feeling positive and optimistic about being old.

That such findings of pessimism and low morale are quite understandable for elderly Hispanics is supported by a number of researchers who have identified many of the severe problems faced by these elders. Santos (in press) emphasizes that economic factors are the major predictors of life satisfaction among the elderly, and therefore he points to the extreme poverty suffered by most Hispanic elderly. A specific problem mentioned by Santos is Hispanics' work-related disabilities that lead to sudden, early retirement. His point is that early retirement means more poverty sooner for the elderly. Santos also cites the economic paradox of old age for Hispanic elderly, wherein they have few earnings and are less able to work and yet they are confronted with more expenditures than in their youth for health problems, special diets, special transportation, and related needs.

A similar argument is found in the observations of I. Cuéllar (in press), who explains that the elderly have a reduced capacity to cope with stress due to less physical strength, less social support, less perceptual ability, and even senility. The sad paradox is that in this time of their lives when they are less able to cope, the elderly are most vulnerable to a host of major stresses (for example, illness, hospitalization, bereavement of loved ones, pain, loneliness, immobility, unemployment, age discrimination, reduced income, and criminal victimization). To these problems, I. Cuéllar adds several that are distinctive for Hispanic elderly, namely, racial prejudice, language problems, exceptionally low income, migration stresses (moving from Latin America and/or rural areas to American cities), and loss of their culture and family supports (see also Cook, 1977).

Both empirical data and the accompanying inferences seem to overwhelmingly indicate that Hispanic elderly are very vulnerable to low morale and mental health problems. Nevertheless, the issue is not so easily clarified. The theoretical arguments forwarded by several authors on this issue indicate that morale is not merely a function of stress, but a function of the relative expectations and the continuity in life experiences among Hispanic elderly. Following from Simic and Myerhoff's (1978) conceptualization of aging as a "career," Velez, Verdugo, and Nuñez (in press) postulate that people throughout their lives accumulate social credits, and then in old age they anticipate a positive return on those credits in the form of warm interpersonal relationships, respect, and support. When there is continuity in the person's life (that is, no disruption of social ties nor disruption of values and traditions), then the elderly person is likely to receive the rewards anticipated. But if there is discontinuity, then the elder suffers "delocalization," comprised of alienation, depression, anomie, and low self-esteem. This discontinuity can assume the form of disrupted social or sex roles, status loss, family disunity, geographical displacement, and/or loss of cultural traditions. The essential point, emphasized by Velez et al., is that Hispanic elderly are greatly at risk of experiencing discontinuity in their lives. For example, the move from Mexico or from the rural life that has been the experience of most elderly Hispanics (Estrada, 1977; Galarza (in press); Peñalosa, 1966) constitutes a significant break with the homeland and customs in which these elders were raised. Szapocznik, Santisteban, Kurtines, Hervis, and Spencer (in press) describe the same problems for Cuban elderly who have suffered a sudden displacement from their homeland and culture. A related problem is the acculturation of the elders' children and grandchildren, wherein they no longer speak Spanish, do not adhere to the old values, and are more socially mobile.

Virtually the same argument is found in Korte's (1978) New Mexico study of morale among elderly Hispanics. Korte likens the maintenance of cultural norms to a "game," wherein the loss of norms constitutes a "loss of game," resulting in depression and alienation for the elderly. The critical element found by Korte was the maintenance of family unity and the accompanying norms of respecting and supporting the elderly. Thus, those elderly Hispanics whose families remained tightly integrated experienced high morale, whereas those whose family relationships were deteriorating suffered depression and low morale. It is significant to note in this regard that the paramount importance of family support for the maintenance of morale and self-esteem among elderly Hispanics has been found by many other researchers (Bengston, 1977; Carp, 1970; Clark & Mendelson, 1969; Laurel, 1976; Sotomayor, 1973; Valle & Mendoza, 1978).

To add another twist to what appears to be a clear-cut issue, even the theory of continuity/discontinuity is not invariably accurate. For example, the important finding of Nuñez (1976) is that discontinuity, in and of itself, does not necessarily lead to depression. Instead, it is sudden, unexpected discontinuities that appear to be the most psychologically damaging. Thus, a retirement that is anticipated and planned for is less traumatic than one that is suddenly imposed by an unexpected physical disability. Similarly, Korte (1978) observes that the great stresses caused by modernization and acculturation are mitigated by these changes and are often gradual, occurring over many years. Thus, a significant morale difference can be anticipated in an elderly Mexican who has lived in the United States for 50 years versus a Cuban elder suddenly leaving Cuba for the United States. This reasoning corresponds to Morgan's (1976) study of widowhood, wherein she found that the expected loss of a spouse due to a prolonged illness allowed the widow time to adjust. But the sudden death of a spouse, she learned, was very likely to cause personal and social disorganization and low morale among widows.

To go full circle in identifying the complexities in the issue of morale, it must be noted that other researchers have found many positive, enjoyable elements among Hispanic elders. For example, Sotomayor (1973) reports that in her sample of Mexican-American grandparents, family unity and traditions were not eroding and, moreover, these elders received love and respect and felt themselves to be active, valuable members of their families. Similarly, Clark and Mendelson (1969) report on the happiness of one elder who felt useful in her family and, most significantly, was very healthy and therefore able to live an active, productive life in her old age.

To conclude, the most basic observation that seems possible is that a number of key factors have been identified as of vital importance to the morale and mental health of Hispanic elders, most notably family unity, maintenance of traditional culture and values (including love and respect for elders), good health, economic resources, and having useful activities to perform. Clearly, all of these factors are, in effect, double-edged swords for the elderly. If they receive the love and support they expect from relatives, are able to remain healthy, and can avoid severe poverty, then they are able to maintain high morale. But if they suffer disruption, discontinuity, or other problems in these areas, then they are most vulnerable to depression, loneliness, alienation, and other forms of low morale and mental disorder.

CONCLUSION

The objective of this discussion has been to provide a brief but comprehensive overview of the Hispanic elderly literature. Embedded within this review, although perhaps not immediately apparent, has been this author's concern for a holistic perspective for examining and understanding the life experiences of Hispanic elders. Thus, the separate discussions, of health, social, and psychological factors were not intended to remain separate in the reader's mind but instead to promote recognition of the complex interactions among these factors (for example, the interrelationship between health, family support, and morale; or the dilemma of barriers to resource utilization creating a vacuum for support if the elder's family relationships are deteriorating).

This concern with a holistic approach for future research echoes the concerns expressed by Ruiz and Miranda (in press) and Miranda and Ruiz (in press) in their recommendations for Hispanic gerontology. Specifically, they call for multiple measurement approaches that recognize the complexities of such key variables as the mental health, age, and culture of Hispanic elderly. In view of the excellent detail and breadth of Miranda and Ruiz's recommendations for research and service delivery, the reader is strongly urged to refer to them. It is hoped that the present discussion has been successful in apprising the reader of the main issues and problems in the field of Hispanic gerontology, thereby serving as a stimulus for more research and services for these deserving elders.

NOTES

1. An in-depth review of Ph.D. dissertations in this field is provided by A. O. Korte (in press).

2. A review of these problems with the literature is provided by Newton (in press) and Newton & Ruiz (in press).

3. Detailed analyses of elderly Mexican-Americans' economic problems are provided by Newton and Ruiz (in press) and Santos (in press).

4. For a concise review of the complex arguments and extensive literature addressing modernization theory in Hispanic gerontology, the reader is referred to A. O. Korte (in press).

5. A more complete discussion of elderly Hispanics' perceptions of aging is provided by Newton and Ruiz (in press).

REFERENCES

Acosta, M. R. Ethnic adaptation by the Hispanic elderly. La Luz, 1975, 4, No. 4, 24-25.

Atencio, T. A. A comparison of the ideological foundations of social welfare and Chicano values. Paper presented at the Symposium on the Chicano Family, Albuquerque, New Mexico, November 1976.

Bengston, V. L. Ethnicity and perceptions of aging. Paper presented at the Conference on Aging, Vichy, France, April 1977.

Bengston, V. L., Cuéllar, J. B., & Ragan, P. K. Stratum contrasts and similarities in attitudes toward death. Journal of Gerontology, 1977, 32, 76-88.

Blau, Z. S. Aging, social class, and ethnicity. Ann Arbor: University of Michigan, School of Social Work, Leon and Josephine Winkleman Lectures, 1978, pp. 1-32.

Carp, F. M. Housing and minority group elderly. Gerontologist, 1969, 9, 20-24.

Carp, F. M. Communicating with elderly Mexican Americans. Gerontologist, 1970, 10, 126-34.

Castro, E. Q., Dehmer, E., Edmond, C. D., Hernández, I., Larios, A. B., Ramos, M. D., Torres, M. S., & Wincowski, R. An exploratory study on the coping mechanisms and utilization of community services among Mexican American elderly living in East Los Angeles. Unpublished Master's thesis, University of Southern California, School of Social Work, 1978.

Clark, M. Patterns of aging among the elderly poor of the inner city. Gerontologist, 1971, 11, 58-66.

Clark, M., & Anderson, B. G. Culture and aging. Springfield, Illinois: Charles C. Thomas, 1967.

Clark, M., & Mendelson, M. Mexican American aged in San Francisco: A case description. Gerontologist, 1969, 9, 90-95.

Cook, K. M. Perceptions of the mental illness of depression among elderly Chicanos. Unpublished Master's thesis, Our Lady of the Lake University, Worden School of Social Work, 1977.

Cooper, T., Simonin, M., & Newquist, D. Project MASP: Health fact sheet. Los Angeles: Andrus Gerontology Center, 1978.

Crouch, B. Age and institutional support. Journal of Gerontology, 1972, 27, 524-29.

Cuéllar, J. B. El oro de maravilla. Unpublished Ph.D. dissertation, University of California, Los Angeles, 1977.

Cuéllar, J. B. El senior citizen's club. In B. Myerhoff & A. Simic (Eds.), Life's career—Aging. Beverly Hills: Sage Publications, 1978, pp. 207-30.

Cuéllar, J. B. Reduction of barriers to delivery of social services. Testimony presented to California State Assembly Committee on Aging, Hearings on Hispanic Elderly, San Diego, November 28, 1979.

Cuéllar, I. Service delivery and mental health services for Chicano elders. In M. Miranda & R. A. Ruiz (Eds.), Chicano aging and mental health. San Francisco: Human Resources Corporation, in press.

Dowd, J. J., & Bengston, V. L. Aging in minority populations. Journal of Gerontology, 1974, 33, 427-36.

Estrada, L. Spanish origin elderly: A demographic survey. Unpublished manuscript, University of California, Los Angeles, Department of Urban Planning, 1977.

Gaitz, C. M., & Scott, J. Mental health of Mexican Americans: Do ethnic factors make a difference? Geriatrics, 1974, 29, No. 11, 103-10.

Galarza, E. Forecasting future cohorts of Mexicano elders. In M. Miranda & R. A. Ruiz (Eds.), Chicano aging and mental health. San Francisco: Human Resources Corporation, in press.

Garcia-Mohr, M. A minority strategy for meeting the nutritional needs of Hispanic elderly. Testimony presented to California State Assembly Committee on Aging, Hearings on Hispanic Elderly, San Diego, November 28, 1979.

Hill, A. O. The Spanish-speaking elderly and vital health concerns. La Luz, 1975, 4(4), 17.

Kasschau, P. L. Age and race discrimination reported by middle-aged and older persons. Social Forces, 1977, 5, No. 3, 728-42.

Keefe, S. E., Padilla, A. M., & Carlos, M. L. The Mexican-American extended family as an emotional support system. Human Organization, 1979, 38, No. 2, 144-52.

Korte, A. O. Social interaction and morale among Spanish-speaking elderly. Unpublished Ph.D. dissertation, University of Denver, 1978.

Korte, A. O. Theoretical perspectives in mental health and the Mexicano elders. In M. Miranda & R. A. Ruiz (Eds.), Chicano aging and mental health. San Francisco: Human Resources Corporation, in press.

Laurel, N. An intergeneration comparison of attitudes toward the support of aged parents: A study of Mexican-Americans in two South Texas communities. Unpublished Ph.D. dissertation, University of Southern California, 1976.

LeBovit, C. The food of older persons living at home. Journal of the American Dietetic Association, 1965, 46, No. 4, 285-89.

Litwak, E. Extended kin relations in an industrial democratic society. In E. Shanas & G. F. Strieb (Eds.), Social structure and the family: Generational relations. Englewood Cliffs, N. J.: Prentice-Hall, 1965, pp. 290-323.

Maldonado, D. The Chicano aged. Social Work, 1975, 20, 213-16.

Manuel, R. C., & Bengston, V. L. Ethnicity and family patterns in mature adults: Effects of race, age, SES, and sex. Paper presented at the Annual Meeting of the Pacific Sociological Association, San Diego, March 1976.

Mendoza, L. Non-kin support networks of the Hispano/Mexicano elderly: Implications for health services research and health services delivery. Paper presented at the Hispanic Health Services Research Conference, Albuquerque, Nex Mexico, September 1979. (a)

Mendoza, L. Integration of community support systems into social policy. Testimony to California State Assembly Committee on Aging, Hearings on Hispanic Elderly, San Diego, November 28, 1979. (b)

Miranda, M., & Ruiz, R. A. Research on the Chicano elderly: Theoretical and methodological issues. In M. Miranda & R. A. Ruiz (Eds.), Chicano aging and mental health. San Francisco: Human Resources Corporation, in press.

Moore, J. W. Situational factors affecting minority aging. Gerontologist, 1971, 11, 88-92.

Morgan, L. A. A re-examination of widowhood and morale. Journal of Gerontology, 1976, 31, No. 6, 687-95.

Morgan, L. A., & Bengston, V. L. Measuring perceptions of aging across social strata. Paper presented at the 29th annual meeting of the Gerontological Society, New York, October 1976.

Newton, F. Issues in research and service delivery among Mexican American elderly: a concise statement with recommendations. Gerontologist, in press.

Newton, F., & Ruiz, R. A. Chicano culture and mental health among the elderly. In M. Miranda & R. A. Ruiz (Eds.), Chicano aging and mental health. San Francisco: Human Resources Corporation, in press.

Newquist, D., Berger, M., Kahn, K., Martínez, C., & Burton, L. Prescription for neglect: Experiences of older Blacks and Mexican Americans with the American health care system. Los Angeles: University of Southern California, Andrus Gerontology Center, 1979.

Nuñez, F. Variations in fulfillment of expectations of social interaction and morale among aging Mexican Americans and Anglos. Paper presented at the annual meeting of the Gerontological Society, Louisville, Kentucky, October 1976.

Peñalosa, F. The changing Mexican American in Southern California. Sociology and Social Research, 1966, 51, 405-17.

Ragan, P. K. Ethnic and racial variation in aging. Paper presented at the 105th annual forum of the National Conference of Social Welfare, Los Angeles, May 1978.

Ragan, P. K., & Simonin, M. S. Social and cultural context of aging: Community survey report. Los Angeles: University of Southern California, Andrus Gerontology Center, 1977.

Reich, J. M., Stegman, M. A., & Stegman, N. W. Relocating the dispossessed elderly: A study of Mexican Americans. Philadelphia: University of Philadelphia, Institute for Environmental Studies, 1966.

Reynolds, D. K., & Kalish, R. A. Anticipation of futurity as a function of ethnicity and age. Journal of Gerontology, 1974, 29, No. 2, 224-31.

Ruiz, R. A., & Miranda, M. A priority list of research questions on the mental health of Chicano elderly. In M. Miranda & R. A. Ruiz (Eds.), Chicano aging and mental health. San Francisco: Human Resources Corporation, in press.

Salcido, R. M. Health advocacy for Mexican American seniors. Unpublished manuscript, University of Southern California, School of Social Work, 1979. (a)

Salcido, R. M. Problems of the Mexican American elderly in an urban setting. Social Casework, December 1979, 609-15. (b)

Salcido, R. M. Health services and the Mexican American elderly. Paper presented at the 7th National Institute on Minority Aging, San Diego, February 1980.

Santos, R. Aging and Chicano mental health: An economic perspective. In M. Miranda & R. A. Ruiz (Eds.), Chicano aging and mental health. San Francisco: Human Resources Corporation, in press.

Scott, J., & Gaitz, C. M. Ethnic and age differences in mental measurements. Diseases of the Nervous System, 1975, 36, No. 7, 389-93.

Simic, A., & Myerhoff, B. G. Conclusion. In B. G. Myerhoff & A. Simic (Eds.), Life's career—Aging. Beverly Hills: Sage Publications, 1978, pp. 231-46.

Sotomayor, M. Mexican American interaction with social systems. Social Casework, 1972, 52, 316-24.

Sotomayor, M. A study of Chicano grandparents in an urban barrio. Unpublished Ph.D. dissertation, University of Denver, 1973.

Steglich, W. G., Cartwright, W. J., & Crouch, B. Survey of needs and resources among aged Mexican Americans. Lubbock, Texas: Texas Technological College, 1968.

Szapocznik, J., Lasaga, J., Perry, P., & Solomon, J. Outreach in the delivery of mental health services to Hispanic elders. Hispanic Journal of Behavioral Sciences, 1979, 1, No. 1, 21-40.

Szapocznik, J., Santisteban, D., Kurtines, W. M., Hervis, O. E., & Spencer, F. Life enhancement counseling: A psychosocial model of services for Hispanic elders. In E. E. Jones & S. J. Korchin (Eds.), Minority mental health. New York: Holt, Rinehart & Winston, in press.

Torres-Gíl, F. Age, health, and culture: An examination of health among Spanish-speaking elderly. In M. Montiel (Ed.), Hispanic families. Washington, D.C.: COSSMHO, 1978, 83-102.

Torres-Gíl, F., & Becerra, R. M. The political behavior of the Mexican American elderly. Gerontologist, 1977, 17, No. 5, 392-99.

Torres-Gíl, F., Newquist, D., & Simonin, M. S. Housing and the diverse aged. Los Angeles: University of Southern California, Andrus Gerontology Center, 1978.

U.S. Bureau of the Census. Current population reports. Persons of Spanish origin in the United States: March 1976. Series P-20, No. 302. Washington, D.C.: U.S. Government Printing Office, 1976.

Valle, R., & Martínez, C. Natural networks of Latinos of Mexican heritage: Implications for mental health. In M. Miranda & R. A. Ruiz (Eds.), Chicano aging and mental health. San Francisco: Human Resources Corporation, in press.

Valle, R., & Mendoza, L. The elder Latino. San Diego: The Campenile Press, 1978.

Velez, C., Verdugo, R., & Nuñez, F. The politics of the aged and the politics of aging. In M. Miranda & R. A. Ruiz (Eds.), Chicano aging and mental health. San Francisco: Human Resources Corp., in press.

White House Conference on Aging. The Spanish-speaking elderly. Washington, D.C.: U.S. Government Printing Office, 1971.

3

SEX ROLES AMONG CHICANOS:
STEREOTYPES, CHALLENGES, AND CHANGES

Melba J. T. Vásquez and Anna M. González

> They say we are nonachievement oriented, inept,
> docile, apathetic, totally without aspirations; we
> allow ourselves to be exploited and physically and
> sexually abused; we are masochistic, self-belittling,
> self-abnegating, subservient, self-sacrificing,
> suffering martyrs; we are passive, dependent,
> possessive, depressive, and neurotic; we are pro-
> ducers of large families, ever fertile, dedicated
> super-mothers with boundless love and nurturance
> for all. They say we are sometimes passionate,
> sexy, voluptuous, dark eyed, hot-tempered beauties;
> other times we are chaste and sexually pure; we
> are "mamacitas": fat women surrounded by five or
> six little brown-skinned children, always cooking.
> This is what they say we are. Is that who we
> really are?

Sex roles in the Chicano* culture and questions about the
psychological nature of Chicano men and women are controversial
issues that are emerging in the social science literature. Various
controversial components of stereotypic sex roles in the Chicano
culture include: first, male dominance, power, and influence
(machismo) and female submissiveness and lack of power and
influence (hembrismo), particularly in conjugal decision making;
and second, male superiority and female inferiority. Based on

---

*The terms "Chicano" and "Mexican-American" are used
interchangeably throughout this paper to refer to individuals
of Mexican origin in the United States.

Rubel's (1966) work, Murillo (1976) described male dominance in this way:

> The husband and father is the autocratic head of
> the household. He tends to remain aloof and independ-
> ent from the rest of the family. Few decisions can
> be made without his approval or knowledge. He is
> free to come and go as he pleases without explanation
> to or questions by other family members. In essence
> the father represents authority within the family.
> All other family members are expected to be respect-
> ful of him and to accede to his will or direction.
> (p. 21)

Thus the father is seen as restrictive and domineering with a neurotic compulsion toward masculinity. Murillo (1976) also describes female submissiveness in this manner:

> The wife-mother is supposed to be completely devoted
> to her husband and children. Her role is to serve
> the needs of her husband, support his actions and
> decisions, and take care of the home and the children.
> In substance she represents the nurturant aspects
> of the family life. Although she is usually highly
> respected and revered, her personal needs are con-
> sidered to be secondary to those of the other family
> members. (p. 21)

The image of the self-sacrificing martyr who does not have any aspirations for self is thus vividly portrayed.

Bermudez (1955) coined the term "hembrismo" to depict the traditional female role which she defines as an amplification of the characteristics that social scientists consider feminine, that is, weakness, passivity, and inertia. Peñalosa (1968) provides a detailed description of the sharply differentiated roles of the husband and wife, which have their basis in the phenomena of machismo and hembrismo. He points out that the machismo and hembrismo sex roles require men and women to behave, think, and feel in rigid predictable, complementary patterns. Women are supposed to be faithful, men are not; women are expected to obey parents, men are not; women are weak, men are strong; women are emotional, men are intelligent.

Male superiority generally has to do with the superior position that men occupy in public life. They command and receive high levels of power, prestige, and status. Women, on

the other hand, occupy inferior positions and their role is ascrib
considerably lower levels of power, status and prestige. Socioeconomic indexes are related to the degree of power an individua
has in American society. Chicanos have among the lowest educational, occupational, and economic levels (Project on the Status
and Education of Women, 1975; U.S. Bureau of the Census, 1978
Attribution of that powerlessness will be dealt with later in this
chapter. While Mexican-American men do not experience the
superiority that nonminority males do in U.S. society, they do
receive higher levels of power, prestige, and status compared
to Mexican-American women.

The extent to which sex role stereotypes occur in the
Chicano culture is not clear. Many of the negative, pejorative
stereotypes have been promoted by social science literature.
The purpose of this chapter is to address some of the interrelate
and complex issues about sex roles among Chicanos, and particu
larly to challenge some of the stereotypes that exist about Mexica
American women.

Four major areas will be addressed. First, sex role stereo
types in the social science literature are identified. Second,
the deleterious effects of stereotyping on Chicanos will be
addressed. Third, studies conducted primarily by Chicano
researchers that provide challenges and contradictions to the
negative stereotypes will be reviewed. Finally, an attempt will
be made to provide a perspective in which to acknowledge variou
changes in which Mexican-American women are involved as they
struggle to obtain equality as women in the family and as minorit
members in the larger society.

SEX ROLE STEREOTYPES IN THE SOCIAL
SCIENCE LITERATURE

Much of the early social science literature concerning
Chicanos has promoted negative stereotypes about origins,
history, identity, and, in particular family patterns and sex
roles. Many of the negative stereotypic portrayals have been
perpetuated by misapplication of a "social deficit" model to the
study of Mexican-American families. That is, social scientists
have assumed that the Anglo norms are ideal and that deviation
from those norms is pathological. Madsen (1961), for example,
contrasts what he describes as the "democratic" family of Anglos
with its concept of male and female equality to the Mexican-
American family, which he describes as maintaining very rigid
sex roles. According to Madsen, the Chicano is the absolute

master in his home, while the Chicana is extremely devoted to her husband:

> She waits on her husband and shows him absolute
> respect, for to do otherwise would be a reflection
> on his manhood. She does not resent her subordinate
> role or envy the independence of Anglo women, since
> her fulfillment lies in helping her husband achieve
> his goals. . . . (1961, pp. 10-11)

Madsen takes male dominance, which Parker and Parker (1979) consider a cross-cultural phenomena, and uses it to attribute pathology in the Chicano family. While male dominance can certainly be pathological in any culture, especially when taken to an extreme, Madsen's ethnocentric perceptions and interpretations have been challenged (Andrade, 1980; Hernández, 1974; Mirandé, 1977).

Misinterpretation of data, impressionistic essays, and generalizations of data for all Chicanos without regard to other important factors such as age, socioeconomic class, generation, and regional location have all contributed to and perpetuated negative myths (Hernández, 1974; Montiel, 1973). Heller's (1966) study depicting Mexican-American women as nonachievement-oriented, passive, and dependent, for example, relies heavily on a study by Kluckhohn and Strodbeck (1961), which is based on a sample of 23 persons in a rural New Mexican community of 150 persons. She concludes that Mexican-American cultural values impede achievement.

The authors, as well as many of their Hispanic female colleagues, have experienced evidence that the negative stereotype of the nonachievement-oriented female as described by Heller continues to be perpetuated. Throughout the authors' higher education, graduate work, and even professional careers, nonminority individuals who maintained those stereotypes repeatedly pointed out that, as achieving Chicanas, they were exceptions, implying that Mexican-Americans are not interested in higher education and achievement in general. It is not unusual for successful, high-achieving Chicano women to hear comments such as, "Oh, but you are different" or ". . . you must be adopted [by an Anglo family]" or ". . . Is one of your parents Anglo?" Rather than acknowledge that the prejudicial stereotype may be inappropriate, nonminority individuals deal with their cognitive dissonance by attributing the success to acculturation or the influential presence of a nonminority person! They do not acknowledge that other variables, such as oppression, may account for the low achievement of Mexican-American women. Zimbardo (1979) points out that prejudice is not only based on beliefs and attitudes formed on the basis of incomplete information but those beliefs are relatively immune to contrary informational input. Contrary information about a Chicana thus makes the individual an "exception."

Fortunately, a growing list of writers have challenged the literature that perpetuates inappropriate perpetuation of myths and stereotypes and pointed out how much of those writings ignore the diversity and heterogeneity among Chicanos. Romano (1968) bitterly critiques the general stereotype concepts of a traditional culture and the image of the nonintellectual Mexican-American promoted by such works as Edmonson (1957), Kluckhohn and Strodbeck (1961), Heller (1966), Madsen (1961, 1964), Saunders (1954), and Tuck (1946). Yet, these works, he states have become authoritative sources on Mexican-Americans and are widely accepted in anthropology and sociology departments in American colleges and universities.

Alvírez and Bean (1976) point out that male dominance is perhaps the characteristic most emphasized in the distorted literature describing family life on Mexican and Mexican-American families. Padilla and Ruiz (1973), in a review of the literature about the structure and function of the traditional Spanish-speaking, Spanish-surname family, describe sex role behaviors, attitudes, and expectations for which they find much agreement among various authors. These include "an authoritarian father and a submissive mother," and "mutual acceptance of the male doctrine of male superiority" (p. 35). Yet, despite the unanimity of this stereotype, Padilla and Ruiz note that very little confirmatory data exist. Mirandé (1977) agrees in his review of conflicting views of the Chicano family by reporting that "despite the absence of hard data, generalizations of the Mexican American abound" (p. 747). Furthermore, he points out that those generalizations present the Mexican-American family in a pathological and pejorative manner.

Murillo (1976) cogently points out the difficulties in describing the traditional Mexican-American family:

> The reality is that there is no Mexican American
> family "type." Instead there are literally thousands
> of Mexican American families, all differing signifi-
> cantly from one another along a variety of dimensions.
> There are significant regional, historical, political,
> socioeconomic, acculturation, and assimilation
> factors, for example, which result in a multitude
> of family patterns of living. . . . (pp. 15-61)

Murillo (1976) and Romano (1968) both critique static concepts that result in the description of an ahistoric people. Therefore, as we identify characteristics and concepts of the Chicano, it is important to remember that all groups are and always have been dynamic and constantly changing. Thus, a view of the "traditional Mexican-American family" may have little or no relationship to reality when historical and other factors are taken into consideration. Murillo also points out that in order to acquire a realistic understanding, one must remember that:

> . . . every value [attributed] to a Mexican
> American person or family should be understood
> basically in terms of there being a greater chance
> or probability that the Mexican American as com-
> pared with the Anglo, will think and behave in
> accordance with that value. . . . in the final
> analysis one must come to know and accept the
> uniqueness of the individual or of a specific
> family. (p. 17)

In summary, social scientists have perpetuated negative stereo-types of Mexican-American men and women (Madsen, 1961, 1964; Heller, 1966). They have depicted men as pathologically dominant and women as pathologically submissive, subservient, and passive. Chicano scholars have begun to challenge the negative stereotypes, pointing out that inappropriate method-ologies as well as distorted interpretations account for much of the inaccurate information. In the following section we will review the more recent studies, conducted primarily by Chicano researchers, that provide more appropriate depictions and per-ceptions of sex role issues among Mexican-Americans.

EFFECTS OF STEREOTYPES OF MEXICAN-AMERICAN MEN AND WOMEN

Social psychologists point out that an individual's self-identity and esteem are partially derived from the cultural feedback of the legitimacy of the person's primary reference groups (Clark & Khatib, 1978; Zimbardo, 1979). Negative messages or denial by a society of the legitimacy of one's impor-tant subgroup memberships—i.e., racial, ethnic, sexual, religious, age groups—can isolate the individual from those who control desired social and material reinforcers within a culture and can result in powerlessness and feelings of incompetence. Chicanas clearly belong to at least two identity groups, ethnicity and gender, which are denigrated by society. The extent to which one accepts the values and messages of the majority group that denies one's own subgroup determines the negative effect on esteem and even performance. Sexism and racism are at times so subtle, however, that it is difficult to innoculate oneself from accepting those messages. Consequently, many Chicano men and women may unconsciously internalize negative self-perceptions.

Mexican-American men and women learn to engage in behaviors prescribed by their culture as well as the society at large through the socialization process. Sex role expectations (that is, beliefs about appropriate behaviors for the two sexes) are thus acquired through that process. Unfortunately Chicano men and women are continuously faced with the negative stereotypes about their sex role behavior and expectations that are perpetuated through language, religion, and the mass media. The internalization of those negative stereotypes, such as the superiority and extreme machismo of males, the submissiveness and nonachievement orientation of females, can result in a limited stereotypic behavioral repertoire. For example, a young man may not feel like a man unless he is dominant and perhaps even abusive of women. A bright woman may be competent but not feel that she can attain her potential and seek higher education. The effects of those stereotypes are therefore deleterious.

Another of the insidious effects of negative societal feedback about one's ethnic group is dissociation through name changes, refusal to speak one's language, rejection of family and peers as well as ultimate turning against oneself. Overcoming the effects that negative stereotyping have on Chicanos is a complex and difficult process. Zimbardo (1979) points out that innoculation against such crippling effects can be accomplished by establishing a sense of pride in one's origins, history, and group identity.

CHALLENGES TO SEX ROLE STEREOTYPES

The literature reviewed in this section is far from conclusive about the various components of sex roles. Implicit in any discussion of sex roles and sex differences is the issue of sex inequality. The issues of male superiority, dominance, status, and power, and the complementing female inferiority and submissiveness are expressions of that inequality and are addressed in various ways.

It is assumed that power and prestige are valued commodities in all societies. Power can be generally defined as the ability to control or exert influence on the behaviors of others (Adams, 1975). Melville (1976) points out some problems in the definition of power in that it can be derived from several sources, including physical force, knowledge, and material wealth. Cromwell, Corrales, & Torsiello (1973) would categorize these as "possessed resources," emphasizing personal attributes and possessions and ideological control which they define as social norms and cultural determinants of who should have power. Most studies that assess the issues of power and influence do so in the context of the Mexican-American family, and it is in this context that controversy exists regarding whether or not Chicanos have power and influence. Differentiation of the context in which a person does or does not have power is an important issue, and will be discussed later in this chapter. Suffice it to say that equality or lack of it between Mexican-American men and women may depend on how one conceptualizes and defines the source of power, that is, from personal attributes and possessions versus social norms and cultural determinants.

MACHO DOMINANCE AND FEMALE SUBMISSIVENESS

Conjugal or marital decision making has been used in many studies as an index of power. Cromwell and Ruiz (1979) critically review four major studies on marital decision making (Cromwell, Corrales, & Torsiello, 1973; Cromwell & Cromwell, 1978; de Lenero, 1969; and Hawkes & Taylor, 1975). They conclude that their review "fails to support the notion of male dominance in marital decision making" (p. 370). Three of the studies analyzed by Cromwell and Ruiz will be reviewed briefly. Cromwell and Cromwell (1978) investigated and analyzed self-report perceptions of dominance in decision making and conflict resolution for an inner-city neighborhood sample of 137 marriages across Anglo, Black, and Chicano ethnic groups. Using six decision-making items, both husbands and wives were questioned separately and results indicated that egalitarianism in conjugal decision making appears to be the norm across and within the three ethnic groups as perceived by both husbands and wives. However, in all groups, husbands attributed more dominance to themselves than wives attributed to them; furthermore, this was most pronounced for Blacks and Chicanos. Cromwell and Cromwell also investigated conflict resolution, which they operationally defined as the perceived outcome of marital conflict when there is disagreement. Once again the investigators reported that the minority couples were experiencing a great deal of conflict concerning decision making. The investigators concluded that the data show more similarities across ethnicities than the theoretical literature and public opinion dictate. However, they also hypothesized, given the discrepancies in husband and wife attribution of dominance and difficulties in conflict resolution of ethnic minorities, that perhaps "normative and cultural expectations are at odds with actual role performance in a changing urban family structure" (p. 757).

Hawkes and Taylor (1975) also found evidence of egalitarianism in conjugal decision making. Using a standardized interview, they explored decision making and action taking of 76 Mexican-American females of migrant families who were from California-operated migrant family camps. Hawkes and Taylor concluded that decisions and actions were shared by husband and wife. They concluded that "dominance-submission patterns are much less universal than previously assumed" (p. 811). They go on to point out that

> Either [dominance-submissive patterns] never existed but were an ideal or they are undergoing radical change. The traditional forces of change—acculturation and urbanization—were not found to be responsible for the results of this study. (p. 811)

Thus Hawkes and Taylor, in addition to presenting data that contradict the notions of male dominance and female submissiveness, additionally propose that while the patriarchal pattern may have been the ideal, it may never have been the norm in reality. Furthermore, acculturation did not seem to be associated with the results of the study.

Cromwell, Corrales, & Torsiello (1973) interestingly avoided ambiguity between norms and actual operating power structure by asking directly for norms. They asked both husbands and wives from Mexico and the United States who should make the final decision in eight areas and who should have the greater influence in four marital areas. While the findings indicated that Mexican husbands and wives exhibit greater patriarchal decision making and influence than American husband and wives, an egalitarian pattern of conjugal decision making and influence was the most common response category for husbands and wives in Mexico and the United States. They conclude that while ideological variables indicated a patriarchal cultural norm for Mexicans relative to Americans, a trend toward egalitarianism was also

evident. In their review, Cromwell and Ruiz (1979), in discussing implications of the Cromwell et al. (1973) study, suggest
the implication that "attitudinal changes have not kept pace with
actual behavioral changes" (p. 365).

Other studies relating conjugal power and decision making
of Chicano families to other variables provide additional and
interesting information. Bean, Curtis, and Marcum (1977)
investigated the effects of conjugal power and decision making
(as well as family size and wife's labor force participation) on
marital satisfaction. The researchers performed a secondary
analysis of the responses of 325 Mexican-American couples from
the 1969 Austin Family Survey, where husbands and wives were
interviewed simultaneously, but in separate rooms. According
to Bean et al. (1977), the findings paralleled those generally
reported for Anglo samples in other studies of marital satisfaction.
That is, Mexican-American husbands and wives were found to be
more satisfied with the affective side of their marriages when
the conjugal power structure is more egalitarian. Interestingly,
both husbands and wives were least satisfied in the wife dominant
group, implying that while satisfaction is most closely associated
with egalitarianism, dissatisfaction is most associated with the
structure farthest from the patriarchal ideology norm, namely,
wife dominance.

In summary, various studies (Cromwell, Corrales, & Torsiello, 1973; Cromwell & Cromwell, 1978; Cromwell & Ruiz, 1979;
de Lenero, 1969; and Hawkes & Taylor, 1975) conclude that
patterns of conjugal decision making in Mexican-American families
fail to support the notion of total male dominance. Other questions
remain, however. Cromwell and Cromwell (1978) conclude that
while egalitarianism appeared to be the norm in conjugal decision
making in all groups, ethnic couples exhibited greater discrepancies as well as more difficulties in conflict resolution when compared to Anglo couples. The authors suggest that normative
expectations may be different from actual role performance for
ethnic couples. Hawkes and Taylor (1975) propose that while
the patriarchal pattern may have been the ideal, it may never
have been the actual norm. Cromwell and Ruiz (1979), in reviewing the Cromwell, Corrales, and Torsiello (1973) study, conclude
that perhaps attitudinal changes have not kept up with behaviors.
Finally, Bean, Curtis, and Marcus (1977) imply that dissatisfaction for both husbands and wives is most closely associated with
wife dominance, which is the structure farthest from the ideal
patriarchal norm.

Other studies utilizing different variables also challenge
the sex role stereotypes of male dominance, or machismo, and

female submissiveness, or hembrismo. Andrade (1980) notes
that one component of machismo has been related to the high
fertility rate of the Mexican-American family. She reviews various
articles (Esparza, 1977; Kay, 1974; Naranjo, 1976; Urdaneta,
1976) regarding family planning and fertility issues and concludes
that machismo may be dismissed as an explanation for the high
fertility rate of the Mexican-American. Variables such as poverty
and social class differences between health care workers and
users are more related to fertility rates than are cultural or
ideological factors or disinterest in regulation of fertility
(Urdaneta, 1976).

In a cross-cultural study examining adolescent perceptions
of conjugal ideological power (norms), Buehler, Weigert, and
Thomas (1974) found that males perceived their father as having
more power than their mother. Samples were from five cultures:
American, West German, Puerto Rican, Spaniard, and Mexican.
Females not only perceived their father as having less power than
males attributed to him, but also as having less power than the
mother. Males not only gave more power to the father, but also
tended to say that the father absolutely had more say than the
mother. Female adolescents tended to report just the opposite.
In this case, power clearly rested in the eye of the beholder.

Various studies, utilizing several variables have challenged
the pejorative view of male dominance and female submissiveness
in the Chicano culture. However, a discrepancy may exist concerning ideological control (that is, the social norms and cultural
determinants of who should have power) and "possessed resources," (that is, knowledge, material wealth, physical force,
labor force participation, and so forth). We cannot conclude,
therefore, that Mexican-American women have egalitarian marriage
relationships. While these do exist, Melville (1980), points out
that they are few and exceptional. What we can conclude is that
the negative connotations of machismo, or the male dominance
concept that has become synonymous with Mexican-American
males and implies powerlessness and submissiveness of Mexican-
American females, does not exist to the extent it has been portrayed. Ramírez (1979), points out that when one speaks of
the negative connotation of machismo, one is referring to male
chauvinism, which is cross-cultural and found in certain portions
of almost all populations. The question that arises is if male
dominance and female submissiveness continue to exist as norms
in the greater societal context, what are the origins and functions
of such sex role differentiations and attributions of power.

MYTH OF MALE SUPERIORITY

The next section of this chapter will attempt to describe the attribution of power and status as they relate to sex roles cross-culturally and to understand the origins of those attributions. Parker and Parker (1979) review the prolific literature that addresses the origins and functions of the institutionalization of sex role differences. Four points are of interest. First, while variations obviously occur in human societies, Parker and Parker conclude that, with very few exceptions, status and prestige are associated with the higher levels of power exercised by males. Even in those societies (for example, Iroquois and hunting and gathering societies, sometimes viewed as egalitarian models) where equality between the sexes is approached, some aspects of women's status are derived from their associations with male kin. The question is, thus, what is the origin and function of the myth of male superiority? Parker and Parker attempt to answer that question by looking at the sexual division of labor. Historically, men's tasks generally

> . . . required qualities such as high-level bursts of strength, danger, achievement motivation, risk of failure, and relatively high levels of techno-scientific training and skill. By comparison, female tasks tended to be more routine, repetitive, and relatively low risk, and did not require as high a mastery of technological skills. (p. 302)

Parker and Parker concluded that women's contributions were quantitatively as great as men's in most societies and qualitatively as important. Thus sexual division of labor did not explain the lower status generally accorded to women.

A third area of interest reviewed by Parker and Parker involves those studies that explore biological sex differences. Parker and Parker categorically rejected the reductionist explanation of the ideology of male superiority or power in social systems as being a direct function of male biological endowment. Females are biologically adapted to reproduce and thus, take a central role in socialization; males are biologically suited for agonistic, exploratory, and strenuous responses, and the data do not indicate superiority or inferiority to either of those biobehavioral functions. Males, in fact, tend to demonstrate more vulnerability to many neurological and other developmental diseases during every stage in the life cycle, including the prenatal stage. Males also exhibit more severe psychological and physical difficulties in reaction to adverse sociocultural conditions (for example, rapid social change, concentration-camp experiences, and so forth). It is generally known that life expectancy is lower for males than for females. The question thus remains, why do men traditionally occupy a dominant position?

Finally, to answer this question, Parker and Parker returned to the examination of division of labor and noted that perhaps traditional male tasks required unequal elements, for example, risk taking, acquisition of skills, and so forth. These greater requirements, coupled with male vulnerability, resulted in a costly male labor supply. The authors hypothesized that society has thus had to offer greater "compensation" to males in order to elicit an optimal supply and quality of male labor. They conclude that the myth of male superiority offered such a cultural reward. It functioned to "psych up" males so they could sustain motivation to achieve in the face of danger or difficulty.

Parker and Parker conclude that ascribing power and status to males thus served an adaptive function for society. They question the current functionality given technological developments that have enabled women to control the number and timing of children, as well as replace needs for high levels of muscular power. The division of labor will continue to overlap as women gain more training and skills because of increased time available to them. Parker and Parker conclude that "the functional aspects of the myth of male superiority are becoming increasingly dysfunctional and even constitute a 'drag' on the ability of society to exploit new sources of energy and creativity" (1979, p. 303).

If we accept Parker and Parker's hypotheses and conclusions, it is clear that male dominance in the Chicano culture has not been too dissimilar from other cultures, and has had adaptive purposes for the maintenance of our society. This leads us to a discussion of implications of changes in the Chicano family.

CHANGES IN THE POWER AND INFLUENCE
OF THE CHICANA

Studies reviewed thus far, those describing the power and influence of the Chicano as well as the review by Parker and Parker (1979), reveal and predict changes in Chicano families such as movement toward egalitarianism in conjugal decision making. Male dominance in the Chicano family has either been exaggerated in the literature in the past, and/or this component of the Chicano life-style is undergoing considerable change.

However, Baca Zinn (1975, 1980) and Mason (1980) refute the notion that changes in the family result from modernization or acculturation, which has been the major framework used to explain changes. In a broader context, Parker and Parker would propose that changes are occurring as a result of technological conditions that result in less need for sex role differentiation, and, therefore less need to reward males with the myth of male superiority. Baca Zinn (1980) looked more closely at specific variables to examine the effect of wives' employment and educational level on conjugal interaction. She found that as women acquired more resources and skills, they achieved greater equality in conjugal decision making without sacrificing ethnicity in other realms of family life. She concluded that power in family decision making rests on economic and other resources, such as acquisition of knowledge and skills.

In an analysis of actos (skits performed by Teatro Chicano), Mason (1980) concludes that the Chicana feminist ideology is similar to Anglo feminist ideology in that the goals of the two movements include egalitarian relations between the sexes and higher status and increased independence for women. However, they differ because while Anglos reject and devalue the traditional feminine role, Chicanas very much value, and in fact, are seeking to enhance the status that has been previously prescribed to that role. Cassell (1977), for example, describes the unspoken rules in Anglo women's consciousness-raising groups where it was permissible to speak of problems with men, but not to speak of good relationships with them; it was socially approved to speak of difficulties and demands of children, but not to speak of the pleasures and rewards of motherhood. In reviewing the Cassell study, Mason concludes that in order to gain equal status and power, Anglo women tended to believe that those roles must be rejected. In her analysis of the actos, on the other hand, Mason observed a commitment to family, community, and ethnic group as well as a desire for equal respect for the contributions and abilities of males and females, including the roles traditionally done by women. The Chicana feminist movement thus ascribes new status to what women have been doing. The Chicana additionally seeks to "open up" her alternatives. Another important difference is that in the Anglo ideology the ultimate group with whom unity is indicated is women; in the Chicana ideology, it is all Chicanos. Baca Zinn (1975) and Melville (1980) describe this prioritizing of the Chicano family and ethnic identity as a reaction to the oppressive elements of American society in regard to minorities. Baca Zinn (1975) states:

> The Chicano family has operated as a mechanism of
> cultural resistance during periods when political
> resistance was not possible. Adherence to strong
> family ties and to a pattern of familial organization
> with distinct sex role differentiation has not indicated
> a mere passive acceptance of tradition. This adher-
> ence has afforded protection, security and comfort
> in the face of the adversities of oppression: it has
> expressed Chicano cultural identity in a society that
> destroys cultural distinctions. (p. 18)

Baca Zinn describes this historical function that the Chicano
family has performed in protecting individuals from the hostilities
of Anglo society as political familism. She believes that the
Chicano movement has fostered a situation in which nationalism
and feminism are both important components.

In summary, male superiority across cultures is a myth
that has served an adaptive function in society. That is, it
served as a cultural reward for men to perform labors that were
more difficult or dangerous than those performed by women.
This myth is no longer functional as change in technological
areas allow for much overlap of labor, and in fact is becoming
increasingly dysfunctional.

In the context of Chicano culture, the male dominance and
maintenance of traditional sex role differentiation may have served
an additional function of protection, security, and comfort in
the context of a larger, oppressive society. A review of recent
literature suggests that either the power and influence of the
Chicana have been misrepresented in the literature, and/or
changes are taking place that result in a move toward egalitarianism. Mexican-American women are involved in dual strategies
of attaining equality as women within the context of families and
as minority group members in the general society. The findings
by Baca Zinn (1980) indicate that these two struggles are highly
interrelated; as women gain more educational, economic occupational and political power in society, they will increase their
power within the family context. Perhaps these changes in resources will ultimately effect the pervasive ideology of male
dominance.

As we seek and acquire more status for the roles of motherhood and the quality of nurturance, we will continue to gain
self-respect as well as power. Melville (1980) cogently summarizes
the hopes and expectations of these authors by suggesting that
Mexican-American women will continue to demonstrate to Mexican-
American men and Anglo-American society that attainment of

power and equality can be acquired without rejection of motherhood or ethnicity.

CONCLUDING REMARKS

Several important questions emerge as we review and integrate the more recent research on the Mexican-American family
and sex roles. There appears to be increasing evidence of
changes in sex roles among Mexican-American families with a
major change centering around the distribution of power in
conjugal decision making.

An important question to address would be the extent to
which Mexican-American couples are experiencing stress by sub-
scribing to certain rigidly defined sex role norms and behaving
differently from what those norms dictate. Which partner is
experiencing more stress? If stress is being experienced by
either or both partners, what are the coping strategies to deal
with the stress? Are they effective?

Other questions that would be important to investigate
emerge when we consider the distinction between sex role behavior and masculine and feminine psychological attributes or
characteristics. Spence and Helmreich (1978) propose that the
sex role concept be restricted to "beliefs about appropriate
behaviors for the two sexes, that is, behaviors that are positively
sanctioned for members of one sex and ignored or negatively
sanctioned for members of the other" (Spence & Helmreich, 1978,
p. 13). On the other hand, masculine and feminine personality
attributes are considered to be relatively stable predispositions
or personality characteristics that are internal properties of the
behaving organisms (Spence & Helmreich, 1978).

The distinction between sex role behaviors and masculine
and feminine personality characteristics is important when we
study Mexican-American sex roles. Gonzalez (1978) found that
more Mexican-American college females were identified as androgy-
nous (that is, highly endorsing both masculine and feminine
personality characteristics) when compared to the normative
sample of Anglo college women. Perhaps the Mexican-American
culture sanctions male and female sex role behavior rather than
masculine and feminine personality attributes. Therefore, an
area to explore is the notion that there are ideological and cultural
differences in sanctioned sex role behavior and defined masculine
and feminine personality attributes.

Actually, as we consider Spence and Helmreich's (1978)
masculine and feminine characteristics that were normed for

Anglo populations, we wonder if Mexican-Americans would make the same distinctions between feminine and masculine attributes.

In the last decade the research on Mexican-American families and sex roles has grown rapidly. The studies are beginning to not only correct the many misconceptions about the sociopsychological nature of Chicanos but also to fill a void in the empirical literature. Hopefully, with the increased sensitivity of researchers to cultural differences we will gain a better understanding of sex roles among Chicanos.

REFERENCES

Adams, R. N. Energy and structure: A theory of social power. Austin, Tex.: University of Texas Press, 1975.

Alvírez, D., & Bean, F. D. The Mexican-American family. In C. H. Mindley & R. W. Habenstein (Eds.), Ethnic families in America. New York: Elsevier, 1976, pp. 271-92.

Andrade, S. J. Social science stereotypes of the Mexican-American woman: Policy implications for research. Paper presented at the American Educational Research Association, Boston, 1980.

Angrist, S. A. The study of sex roles. Journal of Social Issues, 1969, 15, 215-32.

Baca Zinn, M. Political familism: Toward sex role equality in Chicano families. Aztlan, 1975, 6, No. 1, 13-26.

Baca Zinn, M. Employment and education of Mexican American Women: The interplay of modernity and ethnicity in eight families. Harvard Educational Review, 50, No. 1, 1980, 47-62.

Bean, F. D., Curtis, R. L., & Marcum, J. P. Familism and marital satisfaction among Mexican Americans: The effects of family size, wife's labor force participation, and conjugal power. Journal of Marriage and the Family, 39, No. 4, 1977, 759-67.

Bermudez, M. E. La vida familiar del Mexicano. Mexico: Antigua Libreria Robredo, 1955.

Buehler, M. H., Weigert, A. J., & Thomas, D. L. Correlates of conjugal power: a five-culture analysis of adolescent perceptions. Journal of Comparative Family Studies, 1974, 5 (1), 5-16.

Cassell, J. A group called women. New York: David McKay, 1977.

Clark, C. X., & Khatib, S. M. Social change and the communication of legitimacy. Oakland, Calif.: Society for the Study of African Sciences, 1978.

Cromwell, R. E., Corrales, R. G., & Torsiello, P. M. Normative patterns of marital decision making power and influence in Mexico and the United States: A partial test of resource and ideology theory. Journal of Comparative Family Studies, 1973, 4, 177-96.

Cromwell, V. L., & Cromwell, R. E. Perceived dominance in decision making and conflict resolution among Anglo, Black and Chicano couples. Journal of Marriage and the Family, 1978, 40, 749-59.

Cromwell, R. E., & Ruiz, R. A. The myth of macho dominance in decision making with Mexican and Chicano families. Hispanic Journal of Behavioral Sciences, 1979, 1, No. 4, 355-73.

Edmonson, M. Los Manitos: A study of institutional values. New Orleans: Tulane University, Middle American Research Institute, 1957.

Esparza, R. The value of children among lower class Mexican, Mexican American and Anglo couples. Dissertation Abstracts International, 1977, 38, 1397-B. University Microfilms No. 77-17,991.

Gonzalez, A. M. Psychological characteristics associated with biculturalism among Mexican American college women. Unpublished Doctoral dissertation. University of Texas at Austin, 1978.

Hawkes, G. R., & Taylor, M. Power structure in Mexican and Mexican-American farm labor families. Journal of Marriage and the Family, 1975, 37, 807-11.

Heller, C. S. Mexican-American youth: Forgotten youth at the crossroads. New York: Random House, 1966.

Hernández, D. Mexican-American challenge to a sacred cow. University of Los Angeles: Atzlau Publications, 1974.

Kay, M. A. The ethnosemantics of Mexican American fertility. Paper presented at the 73rd Annual Meeting of the American Anthropological Association, Mexico City, 1974.

Kluckholn, F. R., & Strodbeck, F. L. Variations in value orientations. New York: Row, Peterson, 1961.

de Lenero, D. C. E. Hacia donde va la mujer Mexicana? Mexico City: Instituto Mexicano de Estudios Sociales, 1969.

Madsen, W. Value conflicts and folk psychiatry in South Texas. In A. Kiev (Ed.), Magic, faith and healing. New York: The Free Press, 1964, 420-40.

Madsen, W. Society and health in the Lower Rio Grande Valley. Austin: Hogg Foundation for Mental Health, 1961.

Mason, T. Symbolic strategies for change: a discussion of the Chicana women's movement. In M. B. Melville (Ed.), Twice a minority: Mexican-American women. St. Louis: C. V. Mosby, 1980.

Melville, M. B. Twice a minority: Mexican American women. St. Louis: C. V. Mosby, 1980.

Melville, T. R. The nature of Mapuche social power. Unpublished Ph.D. dissertation. Washington, D.C.: The American University, Anthropology Dept., 1976.

Mirandé, A. The Chicano family: A reanalysis of conflicting views. Journal of Marriage and the Family, 1977, 39, No. 4, 747-55.

Montiel, M. The Chicano family: a review of research, Social Work, 1973, 22-31.

Murillo, N. The Mexican American Family. In C. A. Hernandez, M. J. Haug, & N. N. Wagner (Eds.), Chicanos: Social and psychological perspectives (2nd ed.). Saint Louis: C. V. Mosby Co., 1976, pp. 15-37.

Naranjo, M. S. Cross-cultural comparison of social psychological factors contributing to the effectiveness of genetic counseling therapy. Unpublished Master's thesis, The University of Texas at Austin, 1976.

Padilla, A. M., & Ruiz, R. A. Latin mental health: A review of literature. Rockville, Md.: National Institute of Mental Health, 1973.

Parker, S., & Parker, H. The myth of male superiority: Rise and demise. American Anthropologist, 81, No. 2, 1979, 289-309.

Peñalosa, F. Mexican family roles. Journal of Marriage and the Family, 1968, 30, No. 4, 686-89.

Project on the Status and Education of Women. Minority women and higher education, No. 2, Washington, D.C.: Association of American Colleges, 1975.

Ramírez, R. Machismo: A bridge rather than a barrier to family and marital counseling. In P. P. Martin (Ed.), La frontera perspective. Tucson, Ariz.: La Frontera Center, 1979, pp. 61-62.

Romano, O. I. The anthropology and sociology of the Mexican-Americans: The distortion of Mexican-American history (a review essay), El Grito, 2, No. 1, 1968, 13-26.

Rubel, J. Across the tracks. Austin: University of Texas Press, 1966.

Saunders, L. Cultural difference and medical care: The care of the Spanish-speaking people of the Southwest. New York: Russell Sage Foundation, 1954.

Spence, J. T., & Helmreich, R. L. Masculinity and femininity: Their psychological dimensions, correlates and antecedents. Austin: University of Texas Press, 1978.

Tuck, R. Not with the fist. New York: Harcourt, Brace, 1946.

U.S. Bureau of the Census. Current population reports: Persons of Spanish origin in the United States, March 1977. Series P-20, #329, 1978.

Urdaneta, M. L. Fertility regulation among Mexican-American women in an urban setting: A comparison of indigent vs. non-indigent Chicanas in a Southwest city in the United States. Dissertation Abstracts International, 1976, 38, 1507-A. University Microfilm No. 77-18, 607.

Zimbardo, P. G. The social bases of behavior. In <u>Psychology and Life</u> (10th ed.). Glenwell, Ill.: Scott, Foresman, 1979, pp. 624-54.

4

THE MEASUREMENT OF ACCULTURATION

Richard H. Mendoza and Joe L. Martínez

The process of accumulating and incorporating the beliefs and customs of an alternate culture (acculturation) has received considerable attention from the social sciences. One research approach is to study factors that accelerate, inhibit, or are correlated with the process of cultural adaptation. For example, Weinstock (1964) found that in Hungarian immigrants, personality types who had high achievement or goal orientations, hedonistic values, and strong cynical tendencies acculturated faster into the American mainstream society. López (1972), found that physical characteristics also affect the rate of assimilation. Using a sample of male Mexican-Americans, López found that skin color similarity to members of the dominant culture was correlated with acculturation: for males, the darker the complexion of the individual, the greater the tendency would be to assimilate, while for females the opposite was true. Other studies (Burriel, 1975; Martínez, 1977; Ramírez & Castañeda, 1974) found that socioeconomic status, educational level of head of household, community type, generation level, and birth order are all related to cultural adaptation.

A second approach focuses on the psychological manifestations that accompany the acquisition of alternate cultural customs. It is known that rates of transient diabetes mellitus, alcoholism, psychosomatic disorders such as peptic ulcers, and hypertension, delinquencies, suicides, and mortality rates all tend to increase as a consequence of the acculturation process (Hong & Holmes, 1973; Leighton, 1959, Ruesch, Loeg, & Jacobson, 1948).

Others have developed techniques and indexes to measure acculturation. These assessment methods include conformity scales (Campisi, 1947), language usage (Samora, 1956), knowledge of idioms (Sánchez-Baca, 1974), semantic meaning (Martínez, 1977), and cognitive styles (Burriel, 1975; Knight & Kagan,

1977; Mendoza, 1980; Ramírez & Castañeda, 1974). Typically, the techniques employed use Euclidean or correlational models that include multidimensional scaling, factor analysis, discriminant function analysis, canonical correlations, cluster analysis, and multiple regression techniques (Mendoza, 1980; Olmedo, 1980).

In general, very little effort has been devoted to the development of theoretical or empirical models that attempt to describe the dynamic components of acculturation. For this reason, the emphasis of this paper will be to develop an operational model of acculturation.

TYPE VERSUS DEGREE OF ACCULTURATION

Traditionally, acculturation was considered a one-dimensional phenomenon that involved the adaptation of alternate cultural customs. Yet, if we examine the adjustment patterns of American ethnic groups, we find that while some members experience total absorption, others resist acculturation, and still others become eclectics. It would seem, therefore, that a multidimensional model which distinguishes not only between the degree of assimilation but also between the types of assimilation would be useful in describing the adaptation process that we call acculturation.

FACTORS THAT AFFECT TYPE AND DEGREE OF ACCULTURATION

Once exposure to an alternate culture is established, there are a number of elements that one might expect to affect the type and degree of acculturation. For instance, initial attitudes that an individual has about the host or native society can certainly affect subsequent adjustment patterns. One would not expect, for example, immigrant groups who join an alternate culture out of their own volition to acculturate at the same rate, to the same extent, and in the same fashion as socially, militarily, or politically colonized or enslaved ethnic members whose cultures are displaced or substituted by the customs of the dominant alternate society.

Within the immigrant subgroups, one might also expect acculturation differences to occur. An individual who left his/her country out of dissatisfaction with no intention of returning would probably have different attitudes toward the cultural customs of the receiving society than would an individual who left out of economic necessity and who had strong desires to return home. Presumably, permanent groups would be more inclined to display total absorption patterns whereas temporary or transient groups might only incorporate those characteristics necessary for social and economic survival.

Prejudices directed toward an ethnic or racial group by the host society might also manifest themselves in patterns that differ from those of immigrant members that are not subjected to discrimination. Even when a decision to accept and participate in the mainstream society is made, exclusion of immigrants based on religious, racial, or ethnic factors would certainly act to alter the elements of acculturation.

In a similar fashion, the nature of the cultural customs themselves can also affect acculturation. Considering the wide range of cultural practices, it becomes apparent that while some characteristics are compatible cross-culturally, others are not. For example, cultural adaptations involving language usage, food habits, and dress styles are essentially mutually inclusive in that they may coexist in multicultural forms. Thus, one may speak both English and Spanish, eat Mexican and Anglo-American foods, and have Anglo and Mexican friends.

In contrast, cultural patterns that require competitive as opposed to cooperative life-styles or extended rather than nuclear family ties are structurally bipolar or mutually exclusive since the acquisition of one cultural style requires the exclusion of the other.

INCLUSIVE MODEL OF ACCULTURATION

The assimilation of inclusive characteristics is described below by a multidimensional model of acculturation. At one level, the inclusive model delineates between affective, cognitive, and behavioral adaptations. This distinction is important for two reasons. First, some cultural traits tend to be assimilated more rapidly than others. Language usage, dress customs, and technological necessities, for instance, are generally incorporated much faster than abstract or less tangible qualities that involve values, sentiments, esthetic preferences, or attitudes on various socialization practices.

Second, it is also possible that in some cases the cultural pattern of interest may be specific to the cognitive, affective, or behavioral dimensions and require assimilation in only one modality. In such a case, it would be somewhat misleading to conclude that an individual has acculturated to the mainstream society on the basis of the measurement of one cultural trait

such as language. After all, one may speak English out of
occupational necessity, while maintaining traditional Mexican
language, food and dress habits, familial ties, and child-rearing
practices.

At a second level, the inclusive model also distinguishes
between degree of assimilation of dominant cultural practices
and degree of extinction of native cultural customs. This added
dimension is useful if one wishes to explore qualitative differences
in acculturation types. For instance, from assessments made on
assimilation and extinction levels, it is subsequently possible to
establish composite profiles for degree of:

1. Cultural resistance—Active or passive resistance to
dominant cultural patterns as depicted by lack of assimilation.
2. Cultural shift—Substitution of one set of practices
with alternate cultural characteristics as exhibited by simultaneous
assimilation and extinction.
3. Cultural incorporation—Adaptation of patterns that
are representative of both cultural groups as demonstrated by
assimilation without extinction.
4. Cultural transmutation—Alteration of certain elements
of both cultures to create a third and somewhat unique subcul-
tural entity.

The inclusive model is portrayed in Figure 4.1. From
this figure, a number of interesting issues about acculturation
become apparent. First, making use of inclusive indexes to
assess acculturation, as measured by one or all of the components
on Dimension 1, allows the researcher the opportunity to make
qualitative as well as quantitative assessments of acculturation.
For example, if our research goals were to investigate the degree
and type of behavioral acculturation as measured by food habits,
we could assess degree of cultural shift (that is, substitution
of one diet by another), cultural incorporation (that is, assimilation of one diet without relinquishment of the other), and cultural
transmutation (that is, development of food habits that are by-
products of previous practices). Similarly, we could examine
the degree of cognitive acculturation as measured by language
usage, by assessing cultural shift as demonstrated by English
monolingualism, cultural incorporation as measured by degree
of bilingualism, and cultural transmutation tendencies such as
the use of "Spanglish" (that is, combining English and Spanish
vocabulary within the same sentence) or "Pachuquismos" (that
is, slang used among street gangs, or words not readily identified
as being English or Spanish).

FIGURE 4.1

Inclusive Model of Acculturation

**Dimension I
(Modalities)**

	Cognitive	Affective	Behavioral
Dominant Cultural Assimilation			
Native Cultural Extinciton			
Cultural Resistance			
Cultural Shift			
Cultural Incorporation			
Cultural Transmutation			

Dimension II (Types) *(row axis label)*

Where: The last four levels of dimension two represent composite acculturation types derived from the levels of assimilation and extinction.

Note: The last four levels of Dimension II represent composite acculturation types derived from the levels of assimilation and extinction.

Source: Compiled by the authors.

A second issue that becomes apparent from Figure 4.1, is the observation that multifaceted acculturation profiles can emerge across the two dimensions. One may, for instance, be cognitively bicultural by speaking both English and Spanish, display affective cultural shift by having certain attitudes that reflect the sentiments of the dominant culture, and yet be behaviorally unassimilated in terms of food habits and dress preferences. Third, and perhaps most important, the inclusive approach can also be used as an inventory of acculturation.

EXCLUSIVE MODEL OF ACCULTURATION

Assimilation of sociocultural patterns that are nonconvergen may also be investigated in a similar fashion. Like the inclusive paradigm, the exclusive counterpart may also be used as an inventory for assessing acculturation. However, the exclusive approach does not permit extensive qualitative assessments to be made about acculturation types. For instance, if one were interested in acculturation as measured by competitive as opposed to cooperative behaviors, the results might depict a single score on a cooperative-competitive continuum. In this case, the acculturation measure assesses the degree of cognitive, affective, or behavioral assimilation and shift, but not the degree of incorporation, or transmutation.

Nevertheless, one should not hastily abandon the exclusive model for the sake of a more descriptive approach. The assessment of exclusive cross-cultural customs can be used to examine the relative resistance that various cultural norms have to change Unlike the incorporation of inclusive customs that permit an individual to mimic or assimilate the accepted patterns of the mainstream society while maintaining previously held ancestral customs, the adaptation of exclusive cultural norms does not permit the survival of its native counterpart. In the latter case, the immigrant or displaced individual is polarized by the convergent demands of the two cultures. The individual can assimilate and lose a native characteristic or fail to assimilate and face cultural sanction. In the case of the American Indian, an unassimilated child in a classroom setting may share information with a fellow student out of cultural tradition, and yet be punishe by the teacher who views this sharing of information as inappropriate. Furthermore, the use of nonconvergent cultural patterns in the study of acculturation can also be employed to examine the psychological consequences that emerge out of situations that involve cultural conflict. Finally, as a dynamic process, acculturation can be studied across groups and individuals to identify stages that may occur.

In substance, the exclusive and inclusive models should be seen as complimentary paradigms in the study of acculturation With the use of these models, the process of cultural change can be studied as a criterion or dependent variable, and factors such as language proficiency, education level, generation level, sex, and socioeconomic status can be used to predict degree as well as type of acculturation. On the other hand, as an independ ent variable, acculturation types and profiles can be used to examine the consequences of cultural resistance, shift, incorpora tion, and transmutation on learning, alienation, physical, and psychological pathology. It is important to identify situations where acculturation can be used as a dependent or independent variable, so that generation level, socioeconomic status, and other types of demographic information are treated only as correlates, or consequences, rather than as indexes of acculturation.

EMPIRICAL APPLICATION OF INCLUSIVE MODEL

Although it is well established that on most psychological measures Mexican-Americans are more diverse than Anglo-Americans (see Martínez, 1977), little effort has been devoted to describing the nature of that heterogeneity. Making use of the inclusive model as described herein, Mendoza (1980) found considerable differences in the cognitive-style, acculturation types of males and females when measured across generation levels.

For the purposes of assessing cognitive styles, Mendoza (1980) used a modified version of the McKenney and Keen (1974) model. Briefly, the McKenney and Keen inventory consists of a series of tests that measure an individual's problem-solving propensities on two dimensions, information gathering and information evaluation. For our purposes however, only the information evaluation dimension will be discussed.

To assess a person's cognitive style on the information evaluation dimension, an individual is administered two paper and pencil tests that measure the relative skills on each of two opposing modes that are systematic and intuitive. From this evaluation, an individual is described as being either dominant intuitive (that is, having more intuitive skills than systematic skills), dominant systematic (that is, having more systematic skills than intuitive skills), or nondominant with respect to these two information-processing modes.

As expected, it was found that Mexican-Americans were dominant intuitive whereas Anglo-Americans were dominant systematic. Moreover, the variance within groups was much higher for the Mexican-American sample than for the counterpart Anglo-American subgroup, indicating greater heterogeneity among Mexican-Americans.

Due to the high variance exhibited by the Mexican-American group, a secondary analysis that controlled for sex and generation level was conducted to examine the nature of this variance. In accordance with the model, the results revealed a definite trend toward cultural shift and cultural incorporation. For the male

FIGURE 4.2

Multidimensional Scaling Representation of Ethnic, Sex, and
Generation Groups

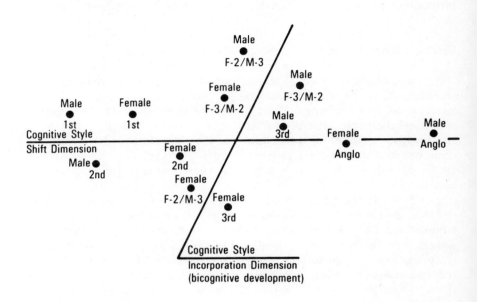

Mexican-American Sample
Male 1st = Male (First generation)
Male 2nd = Male (Second generation)
Male 3rd = Male (Third generation)
Male F-3/M-2 = Male (Third generation by father/
                  Second generation by mother)
Male F-2/M-3 = Male (Second generation by father/
                  Third generation by mother)
Female 1st = Female (First generation)
Female 2nd = Female (Second generation)
Female 3rd = Female (Third generation)
Female F-3/M-2 = Female (Third generation by father/
                  Second generation by mother)
Female F-2/M-3 = Female (Second generation by father/
                  Third generation by mother)

Anglo-American Sample
Male Anglo = Anglo-American Male
Female Anglo = Anglo-American Female

Source: Compiled by the authors.

78

subgroup, first, second, and third generation levels were directly related to cognitive style shift, defined as going from dominant intuitive to dominant systematic. However, for the female sample, first, second, and third generation levels were directly related to cognitive style incorporation, defined as possessing both systematic and intuitive skills. In addition, individuals who were second generation by one parent but third generation by the other parent also displayed cognitive style incorporation patterns.

A graphical portrayal of this outcome is presented in Figure 4.2. First of all, it may be seen that while the Anglo-American groups are located at one end of the cognitive-style shift dimension, the Mexican-American subgroups are dispersed at various points depending upon their respective generation level. On this dimension, generation groups that are closer to the Anglo-American side of the spectrum are dominant systematic, whereas generation groups that lie on the opposite side are dominant intuitive.

Second, the multidimensional representation portrays the extent to which the various subsamples are bicognitive. As evidenced by the cognitive incorporation dimension, Anglo-American males and females show very low levels of bicognitive development as compared to Mexican-Americans. Moreover, within the Mexican-American sample, first, second, and third generation females, and mixed generation members portray the greatest tendencies toward the incorporation of styles that are representative of both cultural groups.

While this study tapped only the cognitive component of the inclusive model, the results demonstrate its descriptive power. Future analyses can make use of this descriptive potential to analyze the relative importance and functional significance of different acculturation patterns to various settings such as employment, learning, teaching, and psychotherapy.

CONCLUSION

We feel that acculturation as a construct cannot be applied generically to the process of cultural change. It is multidimensional in structure and encompasses affective, cognitive, and behavioral adaptations. It is affected by physical and motivational factors, prejudice, degree of contact, and level of participation on the part of the displaced or immigrant individual as well as the host or dominant culture.

In addition, the degree and type of acculturation can also be influenced by the nature of the dominant cultural characteristics. Some customs permit multicultural coexistence (mutually inclusive) while others require cultural shift or absorption (mutually exclusive).

As Herskovits (1937) and Siegel, Vogt, Watson, and Broom (1953) have noted, acculturation should be seen as a dynamic process rather than as an end result. It is a bidirectional phenomenon that can affect change at the individual and group level.

REFERENCES

Broom & Kitsuse, I. The validation of acculturation: A condition of ethnic assimilation. American Anthropologist, Fall 1955, 107, 44-48.

Burriel, R. Cognitive styles among three generations of Mexican American children. Journal of Cross-Cultural Psychology, 1975, 6, No. 4, 417-29.

Campisi, P. J. A scale for the measurement of acculturation. Unpublished Ph.D. dissertation, University of Chicago, 1947.

Cardenas, R. Three critical factors that might inhibit acculturation of Mexican Americans. Unpublished Ph.D. dissertation, University of California, Berkeley, 1970.

Clark, M., Kaufman, S. E., & Pierce, R. C. Exploration of acculturation: Toward a model of ethnic identity. Human Organization, 1976, 35, 231-38.

Dohrenwend, B. P., & Smith, R. J. Toward a theory of acculturation. Southwestern Journal of Anthropology, Spring 1962, 18, 30-39.

Foster, G. M. Culture and conquest: American Spanish Heritage. Chicago: Quadrangle, 1960.

Gillin, J., & Raimy, V. Acculturation and personality. American Sociological Review, 1940, 5, 371-80.

Gordon, M. M. Assimilation in American life: The role of race, religion and national origins. New York: Oxford University Press, 1964.

Herskovits, M. J. The significance of the study of acculturation for anthropology. American Anthropologist, 1937, 39, 259-64.

Hong, K. E., & Holmes, T. H. Transient diabetes mellitus associated with culture change. Archives of General Psychiatry, 1973, 29, No. 5, 683-87.

Kagan, S., & Zahn, L. G. Field dependence and the school achievement gap between Anglo American Mexican American children. Journal of Educational Psychology, 1975, 67, No. 5, 643-50.

Kallen, H. M. Cultural pluralism and the American idea. Philadelphia: University of Pennsylvania Press, 1956.

Knight, G. P., & Kagan, S. Acculturation of prosocial and competitive behaviors among second and third generation Mexican-American children. Journal of Cross-Cultural Psychology, 1977, 8, 273-84.

Knight, G. P., Kagan, S., Nelson, W., & Gumbiner, J. Acculturation of second and third-generation Mexican American children. Journal of Cross-Cultural Psychology, 1978, 9, 87-97.

Leighton, A. H. Mental illness and acculturation. In I. Goldston (Ed.), Medicine and anthropology. New York: International University Press, 1959, pp. 108-28.

López, R. E. An investigation of inter-relationship between skin color, skin color preference, and acculturation-assimilation among Chicano college students. Unpublished Ph.D. dissertation, University of California, Davis, 1972.

Martínez, J. L. (Ed.). Chicano psychology. New York: Academic Press, 1977.

McKenney, J. L., & Keen, P. G. W. How managers' minds work. Harvard Business Review, 1974, 53, No. 3, 79-90.

Mendoza, R. H. Information processing styles: A cross-cultural study. Unpublished Ph.D. dissertation, University of California, Irvine, 1980.

Olmedo, E. L. Quantitative models of acculturation: An overview. In Amado M. Padilla (Ed.), Acculturation: Theory, models, and some new findings. Boulder, Colo.: Westview Press, 1980.

Olmedo, E. L., Martínez, J. L., & Martínez, S. R. Measure of acculturation for Chicano adolescents. Psychological Reports, 1978, 42, 159-70.

Ramírez, M., III, & Castañeda, A. Cultural democracy, bicognitive development and education. New York: Academic Press, 1974.

Ruesch, J., Loeg, M. B., & Jacobson, A. Acculturation and disease. Psychological Monographs: General and Applied, 1948, 292, 1-40.

Samora, J., & Deane, W. N. Language usage as a possible index of acculturation. Social Science Research, 1956, 40, 307-11.

Sánchez-Baca, C. Knowledge of idioms as an indicator of acculturation. Unpublished Ph.D. dissertation, University of New Mexico, 1974.

Siegel, B. J. Acculturation. Stanford, Calif.: Stanford University Press, 1955.

Siegel, B. J., Vogt, E. R., Watson, J. B., & Broom, L. Acculturation: An exploratory formulation. American Anthropologist, 1953, 55, 973-1002.

Smith, W. C. Americans in the making: the natural history of the assimilation of immigrants. New York: Appleton-Century, 1939.

Spiro, M. E. The acculturation of American ethnic groups. American Anthropologist, 1955, 57, 1240-52.

Stonequist, E. V. The marginal man: A study in personality and cultural conflict. New York: Scribner, 1937.

Taft, R. Adjustment and assimilation of immigrants: A problem in social psychology. Psychological Reports, 1962, 10, 90.

Teske, R. H. C., & Nelson, B. H. Acculturation and assimilation: A clarification. American Ethnologist, 1974, 1, 351-67.

Weinstock, A. A. Some factors that retard or accelerate the rate of acculturation, with special reference to Hungarian immigrants. Human Relations, 1964, 17, No. 4, 321-40.

PART II

COUNSELING AND EDUCATIONAL PSYCHOLOGY

5

APTITUDE TESTING, HIGHER EDUCATION, AND MINORITY GROUPS: A REVIEW OF ISSUES AND RESEARCH

Edward T. Rincón

Each year, thousands of college applicants are required to take a standardized aptitude test such as the Scholastic Aptitude Test (SAT) or Graduate Record Examination (GRE) as a condition for consideration in college admissions decisions. Because aptitude test scores strongly influence the choices available to individuals in higher education, considerable importance is generally placed on obtaining the highest possible test score. For many ethnic minority applicants, however, the prospects of obtaining high test scores are typically much lower than for nonminorities. Consequently, fewer applicants of ethnic minority backgrounds are in a position to compete successfully for the opportunities in higher education.

This situation has prompted a considerable amount of debate regarding the fairness of using such tests in college admissions decisions, particularly as it applies to the selection of ethnically diverse groups. In general, studies addressing the fairness of such tests for different ethnic groups have attempted to determine if the test's validity (or accuracy) in predicting subsequent college achievement is similar for the groups in question. In the work of college admissions, however, it is the test score, not the validity coefficient, which remains at the heart of student competitiveness and institutional selection processes. Consequently, it seems equally important to focus on sources of unfairness in the testing environment that lead to lower test scores for ethnic minorities and, hence, decreased participation in higher education.

This chapter will first review patterns of minority participation in higher education since it bears directly on the discussion which follows concerning the controversial role of aptitude tests in the admissions process. This will be followed by a look at the validity of aptitude tests for minority groups and specific factors that may be influencing their level of test performance. It is hoped that this approach will provide a better understanding of how test performance, test accuracy, and minority participation in higher education are integrally related.

MINORITY PARTICIPATION IN HIGHER EDUCATION

In a major effort to extend equal educational opportunity to historically excluded groups, colleges and universities initiated a variety of programs designed to stimulate the participation of Chicanos, Blacks, and other ethnic minorities. Such programs usually included some type of recruitment activities, special financial aid packages, counseling, or supportive course work. Indeed, the doubling of the minority population at college from 234,000 in 1964 to 470,000 in 1970 (Jacobson, 1971) is regarded as evidence that such programs were successful. These figures, however, fail to describe the various shortcomings related to this surge in enrollment.

Compared to Anglo-American (nonminority) enrollments, minority (Chicanos, Blacks, Native Americans, and so forth) college enrollments continue to be severely limited. One study in five southwestern states revealed that only one-third of Chicano high school graduates and fewer than one-half of Blacks enrolled in college compared to 57 percent of the Anglo students (U.S. Commission of Civil Rights, 1971). At the graduate level, Spanish surnamed individuals comprised 1.1 percent of enrollments in Ph.D. institutions compared to 4.4 percent for Blacks and 92.9 percent for Whites (National Board on Graduate Education, 1976).

Sharp inequities are also evident in terms of degree attainment. The National Board on Graduate Education (1976) summarized the following findings for the period 1973-74: Of the total number of bachelor's degrees awarded, 1.2 percent were earned by the Spanish-surnamed, 5.3 percent by Blacks, and 92.3 percent by nonminorities; and of the total number of doctorates awarded, 1.0 percent were earned by Chicanos, 3.5 percent by Blacks, and 87.4 percent by Whites.

The types of institutions and disciplines that minorities select has also been a source of concern. For example, a large proportion of this surge in enrollments for Chicanos (Oliveria et al., 1972) and Blacks (Astin, 1975b) is heavily concentrated in community colleges. Astin is critical of this trend, calling community colleges "educational dead-ins" because they tend to reduce the pool of minority baccalaureates available for advanced training. Moreover, the tendency for minorities to concentrate

themselves in relatively few fields—mostly education and the
social sciences—considerably limits their subsequent employment
prospects (National Board on Graduate Education, 1976).

Finally, for many minority students, attrition becomes a
more vivid reality than degree attainment: only one in four Chicanos who entered college graduated compared to one in two
Anglos (Chronicle of Higher Education, 1975). Degree attainment
at the graduate level becomes a risky proposition for minorities
where approximately half of all doctoral candidates fail to complete
the Ph.D. degree (National Board on Graduate Education, 1976).

In short, while it is true that the absolute numbers of
minority students attending college has increased dramatically,
participation continues to be limited and distributed in a manner
that discourages growth at more advanced levels of training and
subsequent employability.

APTITUDE TESTING AND MINORITY PARTICIPATION

It would be naive to believe that any one reason could
explain the complexities of the problem related to decreased
minority participation in higher education. Numerous circumstances such as inadequate finances, uneven academic preparation,
or reduced motivation can combine to reduce an individual's
overall chances for admission and subsequent degree attainment.

Nonetheless, the one factor that appears to attract more
attention in the controversy regarding limited minority participation is the pervasive use of standardized aptitude tests in college
admissions decisions. Because average minority test scores are
generally lower than Anglo or nonminority scores, such tests
are perceived as the primary means by which the vast majority
of ethnic minorities are excluded from competition in higher education and eventual upward mobility (Samuda, 1975). As Samuda
comments about the original intent of such tests and its impact
on minorities:

> The paradox of aptitude testing lies in the fact that
> it was originally designed to remove the unfairness
> of privilege when access to higher education was
> restricted largely to the professional and managerial
> classes, who could afford to pay the fees for second-
> ary schools that taught the curriculum required for
> college entrance. In practice, though, instead of
> removing class and racial biases from the selection
> process of American higher education, aptitude tests

have tended to reinforce them. Those who have been
the hardest hit by such processes are the students
of ethnic minority backgrounds. (1975, p. 123)

More specifically, critics of aptitude testing argue that
rather than representing actual differences in scholastic potential,
such differences stem from a variety of test-related factors such
as irrelevant test content, unfair testing procedures, heavy
emphasis on verbal skills, or inadequate norms (Flaugher, 1970;
Garcia, 1977; Samuda, 1975).

In contrast, advocates of aptitude testing (Anastasi, 1976)
maintain that the differences in test performance between different
ethnic groups stem from actual differences in cultural environments that should be reflected in test scores. As Anastasi
explains:

> . . . tests cannot compensate for cultural deprivation
> by eliminating its effects from their test scores.
> On the contrary, tests should reveal such effects,
> so that appropriate remedial steps can be taken.
> To conceal the effects of cultural disadvantages
> by rejecting tests or by trying to devise tests that
> are insensitive to such effects can only retard
> progress toward a genuine solution of social prob-
> lems. Such reactions toward tests are equivalent
> to breaking a thermometer because it registers a
> body temperature of 101°. (1976, p. 60)

Anastasi's comments are important in several respects.
First, the assumption is made that aptitude tests have achieved
a level of accuracy that makes their use appropriate in the solution of social problems. As the following section will illustrate,
there is evidence that this assumption can be questioned.
Second, in discussions concerning the fairness of aptitude testing,
the essence of the issue is not that ethnic differences in test
performance should be eliminated, but rather that only those
which are irrelevant to the fair assessment of scholastic potential.
From a practical standpoint, however, the fact that aptitude test
scores consistently provide information regarding individual and
group differences in scholastic ability greatly facilitates the work
of college admissions officers. As the Carnegie Council on Policy
Studies points out,

> . . . it is easier to make policy on what are seem-
> ingly precise and objective grounds; such policies

are easier to explain (although not easy to justify if challenged); such policies tell potential applicants in advance whether they should apply or not; such policies are easier to administer—they can be applied by clerks or by a computer; such policies give admissions officials and others a score card that they can display to trustees, alumni, and other competitive admissions officers. (1977, p. 10)

Thus, as long as the number of college applicants exceeds the number of vacancies, aptitude tests will continue to play an important role in college admissions decisions (Nieves, 1976). This point must not be overlooked in any discussions concerning the fairness of aptitude testing for ethnic minority groups.

TEST ACCURACY AND MINORITY GROUPS

Test Fairness and Minority Groups

Research addressing the fairness of using standardized aptitude tests such as the SAT in college admissions decisions has primarily focused on differences in the tests' predictive validity (or accuracy) between subgroups, and only secondarily on differences in test score levels. Because the principal use of aptitude tests is to predict a future criterion (for example, grade point average), definitive statements about the fairness of such tests are generally held to depend upon evidence of unfair testing practices (Flaugher, 1970), particularly if they continue to predict subsequent performance accurately.

Different models of fairness representing differences in institutional values and desired outcomes have emerged (Nieves, 1976; Olmedo, 1977), each making distinct assumptions and leading to quite different conclusions concerning the selection of minority applicants. Most studies of test bias (or fairness), however, have employed the Regression Model (Cleary, 1968). Cleary states that, "a test is biased for members of a subgroup of the population if, in the prediction of a criterion for which the test was designed, consistent nonzero errors of prediction are made for members of the subgroup" (p. 115). More specifically, unfairness is determined when actual criterion scores are consistently above the predicted scores (underprediction). Overprediction, which is generally not regarded as unfair, occurs when actual criterion scores are consistently higher than predicted scores.

Most research at the undergraduate level addressing the issue of test bias with diverse ethnic groups has been mixed and often characterized by inaccurate predictions for minority groups. Various investigators, for example, have found the SAT to be equally valid for Blacks and Anglos in segregated (Stanley & Porter, 1967) and integrated (Cleary, 1968) institutions. Others, however, have found significant differences in the predictive systems employed (Kallingal, 1971; Pfeifer & Sedlacek, 1971; Temp, 1971). The use of a single regression equation has also resulted in overpredictions and underpredictions of college grade-point average for Chicanos (Brelund, 1978; Goldman & Richards, 1974; Goldman & Hewitt, 1976). Moreover, the SAT was found to contribute only marginally to the prediction of college grades for Blacks (Astin, 1975a; Davis & Temp, 1971) and Chicanos (Goldman & Hewitt, 1976; Lowman & Spuck, 1975).

Comparable research has yet to emerge for minority students at the graduate level (Nieves, 1976). Various circumstances that have mitigated against comparative validity studies include the small number of minorities admitted to graduate institutions and the difficulties encountered in coordinating projects at such institutions. For most students, though, the validity of the GRE has been described as modest, having median correlations from as low as .14 to .48 across a variety of success criteria and disciplines (Willingham, 1973). Hence, it is likely that the accuracy of the GRE in predicting graduate achievement for minority students is not much better than the accuracy of the SAT at the undergraduate level.

The significance generally given to such inaccuracies merits further discussion. Recall that according to Cleary's (1968) definition of test bias, overpredictions are not considered evidence of bias. Because overpredictions result in more admissions for minority applicants, it is thought that this type of inaccuracy "unduly favors" minority candidates (Flaugher, 1970). In the strictest sense of the word, however, overpredictions must still be regarded as a form of inaccurate and, hence, unfair, assessment whose effects are not necessarily favorable for minority students. As Goldman asserts:

> (1) It can be very demoralizing for individuals to be selected for college admission by what may amount to caprice; (2) persistent overprediction may be equated with persistent under-achievement and, therefore, reinforce stereotypes of black inferiority within the black student body; and (3) selection by an inaccurate method can preclude the use of

a better selection method which might select the
successful students in the subgroup. (1973, p. 208)

The central concern about overpredictions is that they
contribute unnecessarily to the underachievement and attrition
of minority students by admitting those who are not expected to
perform adequately. The fact that only one in four Chicanos
who entered college graduated compared to one in two Anglos
(Chronicle of Higher Education, 1975) illustrates the potential
disservice that inaccurate predictive systems can have for minority
applicants and the institutions that they attend.

Given the importance of overpredictions and the frequency
with which they are reported for minority students, is there any
reasonable hope for improvement? There are several reasons to
doubt that any improvement is likely in the near future. Willingham (1973), for example, expresses a general pessimism about
the feasibility of improving the predictive validity of tests since
the range of ability is quite narrow, particularly at the graduate
levels. In this regard, a few studies have noted considerably
lower test variances for Blacks (Astin, 1975 a & b; Dittmar,
1977) and Chicanos (Dittmar, 1977) when compared to Anglos.
Ghiselli (1964) has illustrated that differences in predictor variances between groups can reduce the predictor's reliability estimate and predictive validity. In short, differences in predictive
validity among ethnic groups may stem in part from prior differences in test variances or range of talent.

Another view maintains that overpredictions may result
from the use of first-year grade-point averages for minority
groups (Nieves, 1976). Nieves argues that overpredictions are
likely since minority students generally obtain higher grades
after the first year of either undergraduate or graduate programs. Hence, little improvement can be expected unless success
criteria are extended beyond the first year for minority students.

Finally, Cleary (1968) maintains that overpredictions are
unavoidable when two groups with substantial differences in
average scores are compared, suggesting that "the real problem
is the score differential and the argument should return to that
particular focus" (Nieves, 1976, p. 6).

In view of the multiple problems associated with investigations concerning the validity of aptitude tests for diverse ethnic
groups, Nieves's suggestion is consistent with this author's
belief that perhaps greater progress on the issue of test fairness
can be made if more attention is devoted to an examination of
the factors that contribute toward ethnic differences in test
performance. Indeed, research activity in this area has not

been substantial, possibly because questions concerning the issue of test bias have too frequently relied on validity studies to provide the answers. As Flaugher has pointed out, ". . . the test administration environment can have an influence on test performance; there is potentially a very real source of differential and hence, inequitable, influence on test scores" (1970, p. 18).

Accordingly, the following section will highlight relevant areas of research that provide an understanding of how differences in the testing environment as well as individual characteristics can contribute toward differential test performance among subgroups.

FACTORS RELATED TO DIFFERENTIAL TEST PERFORMANCE

As many individuals can attest, taking an aptitude test for college admission can be a very unpleasant experience. How well one performs on such tests can have a tremendous influence on the choices available in higher education in terms of major, type of institution, and competitive scholarships. Because higher test scores are generally associated with better choices, examinees are particularly motivated to maximize their performance on such tests. This is not to suggest, however, that other criteria besides test scores are unimportant in the admissions process. Rather, as McClelland pointed out:

> Admissions officers have protested that they take
> other qualities besides test achievements into account
> in granting admission, but careful studies by Wing
> and Wallach (1971) and others have shown that this
> is true only to a very limited degree. (1973, p. 1)

As McClelland appears to be suggesting, the bottom line in college admissions is still high aptitude test scores.

Not all applicants, however, are capable of demonstrating their full potential under such stressful conditions. A number of factors, either personal or related to the test environment, can inadvertently interfere with adequate performance on standardized aptitude tests. This may be especially true for ethnic minority groups whose prior acculturation and socialization experiences have resulted in the development of skills or attitudes that are not congruent with standard testing practices. Accordingly, an attempt will be made in this section to focus on specific areas of research that have some bearing on this problem.

Language

The fact that many ability measures are heavily loaded verbally suggests that familiarity with the language of the test is essential for adequate performance (Samuda, 1975). This is especially true of certain ethnic minority groups who may be linguistically different as in the case of Chicanos. Numerous attempts have been made to reduce or eliminate the importance on language skills including the use of visual stimuli (pictures, drawings, diagrams), numerical tasks, spatial tests, and the minimization of written or spoken language. Tests that incorporate such methods are commonly referred to as "culture-free" or "culture-fair." Reviews of the efficacy of such measures in the assessment of minority groups have shown, to the surprise of many, that ethnic differences on nonlanguage tests are frequently larger than on language measures (Anastasi, 1976; Flaugher, 1970; Samuda, 1975). Such nonverbal measures presumably require skills that are more characteristic of middle-class Western cultures, such as abstract thinking processes and analytic cognitive styles (Anastasi, 1976). In summarizing the research in this area, Samuda concludes:

> It is the consensual opinion of psychometricians and psychologists that culture-free or culture-fair tests have proved disappointing and have fallen short of their goals, for minority students have been shown to perform, if not more poorly, at least just as badly as they do on conventional intelligence measures. (1975, p. 142)

Thus, the history of the culture-fair movement aptly illustrates that most if not all forms of assessment are ultimately culture-bound. More importantly, it points to the need for more careful examination of the potential bias that may exist in currently used measures of quantitative ability or other non-language measures for minority groups.

Prior Course Work

For various reasons, many students come out of high school with uneven academic skills. Differences in career goals, for example, lead some students to pursue college preparatory course work while others opt for vocationally oriented programs. Such differences in preparation can have notable effects on aptitude test performance, particularly in the quantitative areas where advanced training or activity is frequently limited.

For example, Ekstrom (1979) reports that studies conducted by the Educational Testing Service revealed that most of the variability in male-female score differences on the SAT Mathematical subtest (SAT-M) is attributable to differences in the number of years of high school mathematics taken by both sexes. Also, the number of types of mathematics courses taken by males and females was found to explain most of the sex differences in quantitative aptitude test scores for high school juniors (De Wolfe, 1977).

Pike (1978) maintains that although the mathematical skills required to answer the SAT Mathematics questions is intentionally limited to ninth or tenth grade content, mathematics course work beyond that level serves as a review and facilitates answering such items. As Pike suggests, ". . . one way to increase ones' mathematical aptitude as measured by the SAT-M is to take additional courses in that subject matter area" (1978, p. 50).

Because considerably fewer minorities than nonminorities enroll in college (U.S. Commission on Civil Rights, 1971), it is likely that minorities enroll less frequently in college preparatory course work than nonminorities. In one study, it was noted that compared to Anglo high school juniors, Chicanos enrolled in virtually no mathematics courses beyond the basic courses required of all students (Rincón, 1979).

Clearly, research is needed to determine if the relationship between course work and test performance is applicable for different ethnic groups as well. In the meantime, research suggests that ethnic minority students might do well to take more mathematics courses as one way to improve their quantitative test performance.

Short-Term Instruction

As admissions criteria at colleges and universities become increasingly competitive, many examinees are turning to "coaching" schools or other forms of short-term instruction in an effort to improve their aptitude test scores. As used in Pike's (1978) review of the literature, short-term instruction refers to ". . . attempts to improve test scores by means of a relatively short period of instruction; relatively short, that is, when compared to the amount of time generally considered necessary for any substantial change in the ability or knowledge in question" (pp. 4-5). Although the structure of such programs varies, typical activities include content review, practice on sample test questions, familiarity with different item formats, and testwiseness. Implicit in these attempts is the expectation that the individual will be at an "improved state of readiness" to determine his/her full potential aptitude as a result of such instruction.

Concern has been repeatedly raised by test developers concerning this trend that the credibility and validity of standardized aptitude tests would be threatened if test scores, which are presumed to measure stable attributes developed over a long period of time, could be easily raised in a relatively short period of time (Nieves, 1976). This would have the effect of eliminating the tests' ability to distinguish between applicants. In contrast, Pike (1978) argues that test validity may actually be improved by providing individuals instructional activities that will allow them to demonstrate their full potential aptitude.

Earlier studies reviewed elsewhere on the effects of coaching (College Entrance Examination Board, 1968) that were completed during the 1950s concluded that overall score gains due to coaching were not sufficient to justify having students invest time in instruction to enhance their test scores. Most students involved in these studies, however, were more advantaged and better prepared to do their best on the SAT compared to current high school candidates. Further, for most studies reporting no differential gains or negative results, instruction was generally brief, relatively uncontrolled, gave little attention to mathematical review, and emphasized only general testwiseness (Pike, 1978).

In comparison, more recent studies reviewed by Pike (1978) reveal average score gains for coached groups on both the SAT Mathematics (SAT-M) and Verbal (SAT-V) subtests that were statistically and practically meaningful, ranging from approximately 43 to 122 points. Interestingly, the popular notion that the verbal subtest is "impervious to change" was challenged by these studies since in some instances SAT-V gains were strongly equivalent to those observed for the SAT-M.

Pike points out that the studies that found significant gains due to instruction differed from the studies that did not because they involved more hours of instruction, were more controlled, incorporated deliberate mathematics instruction, taught specific and general testwiseness, and used students that were at neither extreme of test preparedness or test sophistication. As Pike (1978, p. 61) asserts:

> This difference between comparatively passive, unfocused study and active study directed at specific skills runs counter to the common feeling represented by French and Dear's (1959) concluding comments that rather than seeking coaching, an eager College Board candidate ". . . would probably gain at least as much by some review of mathematics on his own and by the reading of a few good books." (p. 329)

Pike's review provides a considerable amount of provocative information concerning the susceptibility of the SAT to short-term instruction as well as an analysis of specific test components that vary in their "coachability." A specific shortcoming of the studies reviewed, though, is that they provide little additional information concerning which kinds of examinees would be most likely to profit from such instruction. For example, would the same instructional program result in similar gains for Chicanos and Blacks, males and females, low anxious and high anxious individuals? Conversely, for which of these groups is instruction likely to hinder performance? Clearly, the generality of gains related to short-term instruction has not been adequately explored Nonetheless, the review provides critical information that may be useful in the design of similar studies focusing on minority-majority differences in aptitude test performance.

Testwiseness

Although efforts are generally made to include testwiseness as part of short-term instructional activities, it deserves additional consideration since it is not directed at test content per se but at test-taking skills or knowledge that will permit individuals to show their abilities to their best advantage (Pike, 1978).

In his recent review of testwiseness studies, Pike (1978) distinguishes between three forms of testwiseness. The first type is guessing, which is defined as answering a test item in the absence of uncertainty. Guessing can be blind (or random), spurious (or hunched-based), or informed probabilistic (based on partial information). Contrary to popular thinking, Pike maintains that guessing is necessary for appropriate responding to the SAT. Like many situations confronting individuals, he argues, at some point everyone is called upon to make an "educated guess" based on partial information. This is particularly true of the SAT or similar tests of ability that generally include numerous questions at the middle range of difficulty level for examinees. It follows that over a set of items, an individual receives partial credit for partial information.

Individuals vary in their willingness to guess and this tendency is further influenced by a variety of factors including the directions for guessing given to examinees, personal characteristics (self-assurance, aggressiveness, motivation to do well, or indifference about doing well), and the speed of a test (Goldman, 1971). In order to reduce score differences resulting from individual variation in guessing, a standard guessing penalty or correction formula is often imposed. Interestingly, this practice has resulted in some unusual consequences. As Pike (1978) explains,

Ironically, as Slakter (1968a) has noted, research
has shown that even when there is a penalty for
guessing, most examinees would do better if they
did more guessing. He elaborates the point in another
article (1968b), where he notes that the scoring
penalty directions tend to influence most of those
students who are already reluctant to guess, resulting in the guessing penalty becoming, in effect,
a penalty for not guessing. (p. 28)

An alternative to the penalty for guessing has involved
the use of the "rights only" scoring procedure that usually requires examinees to answer all test items (Goldman, 1971). However, forcing examinees to answer all items may also decrease
their scores since differential performance has been observed
according to the particular item format being answered (Pike &
Flaugher, 1970).

The second type of testwiseness is known as risk-taking
behavior. Assuming a given level of knowledge on a test item,
examinees will differ in their tendency to guess despite the
directions given. As might be expected, examinees low in risk-
taking behavior are likely to be penalized on test performance
(Slakter, 1969).

Finally, the third aspect of testwiseness that is also related
to guessing is the issue of answer changing. In summarizing
other reviews of studies on answer changing, Pike (1978, p. 31)
reports the following conclusions:

1. Most examinees express the belief that it does not pay
to change answers.
2. Most examinees, nevertheless, do change answers,
but typically on only about 4 percent of the questions.
3. In fact, it generally does pay to change answers.
Typical findings are that there are about two favorable changes
for every unfavorable change.
4. Gains drop off as items get relatively more difficult.
5. Higher scoring examinees tend to benefit more from
answer changing than do lower scoring ones.

In summary, it is clear that testwiseness comprises a set
of skills that are essential to adequate performance on aptitude
tests and other tests of ability. Indeed, because minority
individuals may already perceive their probability of successful
performance to be quite low, they may elect to be more cautious
or less risky, thereby influencing the frequency and quality of

the guessing and answer changing that occurs. Thus, unless special efforts are made to share these "unwritten rules" with minority students, it is likely that their test performance will continue to remain unchanged.

ANXIETY AND INTELLECTUAL FUNCTIONING

Largely because the testing process monitors access to virtually all facets of our societal structure, considerable tension and anxiety has come to be associated with the failure to meet the rigorous standards defined by such tests, particularly in the academic area. Anxiety and academic performance are increasingly negatively related during the elementary school years (Kirkland, 1971; Ruebuch, 1963; Phillips, Martin, & Meyers, 1972), resulting in poor performance on IQ and achievement tests, grade repetition, and lower grades (Hill, 1971). The relationship is cumulative during the high school and college years, covering all ranges of intellectual functioning (Ruebuch, 1963) and resulting in high dropout rates due to academic failure (Spiegelberger, 1962). In general, high anxiety associated with academic competition is not advantageous.

Reviews of the anxiety literature, however, point to the complex nature of this phenomenon, varying in levels for different groups and influencing intellectual functioning in different ways (Kirkland, 1971; Wine, 1971; Sarason, 1960). For example, high anxiety is generally associated with females, low ability, and low socioeconomic status. More importantly, specific variations in testing procedures have been shown to influence differentially the performance of high and low anxious individuals. For instance, decrements in performance for high anxious individuals are more likely on tasks that include ego-involving instructions; do not provide memory supports; are complex; are unfamiliar; and are highly evaluative or testlike. Conversely, reversal of these procedures has been shown to reduce performance differences between high and low anxious individuals.

Although anxiety level has been shown to vary with ability level, sex, and socioeconomic status, surprisingly few anxiety theorists have explored the generality of this construct for different ethnic groups. Intuitively, one could speculate that depressed social status, which is characteristic of minority groups, increases one's vulnerability to stress. As Schacter (1969) suggests, high anxiety is characteristic of socially isolated groups. That social isolation has become a way of life for ethnic minorities is evidenced by higher rates of unemployment (Poston

& Alvirez, 1976), frequent encounters of prejudice and discrimination (Padilla & Ruiz, 1973) and overrepresentation in classes for the mentally retarded (Mercer, 1976).

Several studies confirm the relationship between ethnic minority status and anxiety level. Higher anxiety scores have been reported for Chicano (Glenn, 1969) and Black school children (Barabasz, 1970) when compared to Anglo-Americans. Similarly, others have noted a tendency for lower-class minority status children to report higher levels of anxiety than other lower-class children (Phillips, 1966; Tseng & Thompson, 1969). One study at the college level, however found no differences in level of test anxiety between Black and Anglo-American students (Hall, 1975).

There are at least two important implications that anxiety research has for the assessment of minority aptitude test performance. First, it provides a theoretical framework with an extensive research base which can facilitate the identification of factors in the testing environment that interact with individual characteristics to produce differential test performance. Second, it enables the investigation of within-cultural-group differences in test performance in addition to between-cultural-group differences, a rather frequently ignored consideration. Indeed, there may be reason to doubt that individuals within a cultural group are behaviorally homogeneous, particularly as it concerns test-taking behavior. Lastly, it would be particularly useful to determine if the anxiety construct has any predictive value beyond that available through test scores in reducing minority attrition rates in higher education.

TEST SPEEDEDNESS

One variation in testing procedure that has been identified as a specific source of evaluative stress for ethnic minorities is test speededness (Anastasi & Cordova, 1953; Evans & Reilly, 1972; Wrightstone, 1963). Tests employing time limits are regarded as specifically stressful to ethnic minorities because they introduce a standard of performance that may be culturally inappropriate. This is somewhat analogous to the findings that high test anxious individuals, who generally work more slowly and more cautiously, perform significantly better in situations that permit them to work without the constraints of time limitations (Ruebuch, 1963; Wine, 1971). Acknowledging their failure to demonstrate their ability, ethnic minorities attempt to shorten the period of discomfort by making random responses, guessing blindly, or leaving the examination site prematurely (Evans & Reilly, 1972; Khan, 1968).

In addition to being a method by which to standardize testing procedures, most tests of ability or intelligence incorporate speed instructions as a matter of administrative convenience. This serves to discourage the slow test taker from taking lengthy periods of time to complete the test. Speed instructions, however, may have different cultural meanings. Klineberg has illustrated that speed is basically a culturally oriented concept. As he explains:

> The attitude toward speed varies greatly in different cultures and not all peoples will work on the tests with equal interest in getting them done in the shortest time possible. Peterson and his associates (1925) have noted this relative indifference to speed among Negroes and the writer found that the injunction to "do this as quickly as you can" seemed to make no impression on the Yakima reservation in the state of Washington. (1935, p. 159)

Further support for Klineberg's position is provided by findings of differences in the concept of time (or time orientation) among Anglo-Americans, Native Americans, and Spanish-American (Roberts & Greene, 1971). Shannon (1976) also observed that Chicanos are less likely to relate achievement to the passage of time.

Assuming that test speededness represents a specific source of bias in testing procedure for ethnic minorities, it seems reasonable to expect that a more accurate assessment of their underlying abilities might be accomplished by eliminating or placing less emphasis on time limits during the testing situation. A series of studies have explored the effects of differently speeded aptitude tests during regular national administrations (Evans & Reilly, 1972; Evans & Reilly, 1973; Reilly & Evans, 1974). Test speededness is generally defined according to criteria established by Swineford (1956) which stipulate that a test may be considered unspeeded if: first, virtually all candidates reach 75 percent of the items, and second, at least 80 percent of the candidates respond to the last item.

Evans and Reilly (1972) administered a specially constructed speeded (40 minutes, 35 items) and unspeeded (40 minutes, 27 items) form of a reading comprehension test to "regular center" and "fee-free" (predominantly Black) Law School Admission Test (LSAT) candidates. The speeded form was found to be more

speeded for the fee-free candidates than for the regular center
candidates with a larger difference in scores for the fee-free
group between the speeded and unspeeded versions. A similar
approach by Evans and Reilly (1973) compared minority (Blacks)
and majority performance on a special quantitative section of the
Admission Test for Graduate Study in Business (ATGB). It was
found that raising or lowering the time limits appeared to have
little effect in changing score levels between ethnic groups.
However, a substantial proportion of dropouts (20 percent)
occurred somewhat earlier for the Black group than for the
White group. Finally, Reilly and Evans (1974) administered a
reading comprehension section of a national academic aptitude
test to Black, White, Chicano, and Oriental college seniors under
30-minute and 40-minute time limits. Although increasing the
time allowed to complete the section had a slightly beneficial
effect for all candidates, this effect was not differential among
the various groups identified.

Last, in what may represent one of the few studies examining the role of test anxiety on speededness-related differences
in aptitude test performance, Rincón (1979) administered the
quantitative subtest of the School and College Ability Tests
(SCAT) to Chicano and Anglo-American high school juniors under
speeded (regular 20-minute time limit) and power (40-minute
time limit) testing conditions. In addition, a measure of test
anxiety was obtained from subjects prior to testing in order to
examine the relationship of this personality dimension to
speededness-related differences in test performance.
The main conclusions that emerged were as follows:

1. For Anglo-Americans, higher levels of test anxiety
uniformly resulted in lower test performance regardless of time
condition, while higher test performance was associated with
lower levels of test anxiety.

2. For Mexican-Americans in the power condition, the
relationship between test anxiety and test performance was
similar to the relationship for Anglo-Americans above.

3. For Mexican-Americans in the speed condition, test
performance and test anxiety were curvilinearly related; that
is, at higher levels of test anxiety increases in anxiety were
associated with higher test performance, but at lower levels of
anxiety increases in anxiety were associated with decreases in
test performance. The lowest performance was noted at the
middle range of test anxiety level.

The findings illustrate the importance of examining within-
cultural-group differences in test behavior. Indeed, if between-

group differences in test performance would have been the only concern, it might have been concluded that test speededness was not a prominent factor in test performance. On the contrary, although speededness had no significant effect on the performance of Anglo-Americans, it was shown to be very important for the performance of Mexican-Americans: speededness was detrimental at the lower range of test anxiety but beneficial as test anxiety level increased. In short, statements concerning the effects of test speededness between groups should be qualified by considera tions regarding the potential variation within groups. Our under- standing of ethnic group differences in test performance should not depend entirely on distinctions concerning ethnic group membership.

SUMMARY

This chapter has touched on patterns of minority participa- tion in higher education with specific attention given to the manne in which aptitude test scores influence this participation. The accuracy of aptitude tests in predicting minority college achieve- ment has been discussed, concluding that although test scores greatly facilitate the admissions process, inaccuracies in the form of overpredictions can potentially encourage higher minority attrition rates and underachievement. In recognizing that little improvement in the validity of such measures can be expected for minority groups, attention needs to be directed to several factors that can potentially influence test performance for differ- ent subgroups. These include language, prior course work, short-term instruction, testwiseness, anxiety, and test speeded- ness. As has been noted, each of these factors has considerable promise for research efforts directed at identifying and eliminatin potential sources of unfairness in testing practices for ethnic minority groups.

As a final note, the author wishes to explain that no deliberate effort was made to exaggerate the importance of standardized aptitude testing nor to suggest that students should become unduly concerned with competitive tactics. Rather the intent was to illustrate that aptitude test performance can vary as a function of other factors besides one's ability level. If it can be demonstrated that the knowledge gained by measuring such factors is important in predicting subsequent achievement, then perhaps test scores should reflect their influence. Other- wise, concerted efforts must be made to minimize or eliminate their respective influences from aptitude test scores.

REFERENCES

Anastasi, A., & Cordova, F. A. Some effects of bilingualism upon the intelligence test performance of Puerto Rican children in New York City. Journal of Educational Psychology, 1953, 44, 1-19.

Anastasi, A. Psychological testing. New York: Macmillan, 1976.

Astin, A. W. Preventing students from dropping out. San Francisco: Jossey-Bass, 1975. (a)

Astin, A. W. The myth of equal access in public higher education. Atlanta: Southern Education Foundation, 1975. (b)

Barabasz, A. F. Galvanic skin responses and test anxiety among Negroes and Caucasians. Child Study Journal, 1970, 1, 33-35.

Brelund, H. M. Population validity and college entrance measures. Research Bulletin 78-79. Princeton, N.J.: Educational Testing Service, 1978.

Carnegie Council on Policy Studies in Higher Education. Public policy and academic policy. In Selective Admissions in Higher Education. San Francisco: Jossey-Bass, 1977.

Chronicle of Higher Education. 11, No. 7, 1975.

Cleary, T. A. Test bias: Prediction of grades of Negro and white students in integrated colleges. Journal of Educational Measurement, 1968, 5, 115-24.

College Entrance Examination Board. Effects of coaching on Scholastic Aptitude Test scores. New York: College Entrance Examination Board, 1968.

Davis, J. A., & Temp, G. Is the SAT biased against Black students? College Board Review, Fall 1971, No. 81, 4-9.

De Wolfe, V. A. High school mathematics preparation and sex differences in quantitative abilities. EAC Report 77-7, University of Washington, June 1977.

Dittmar, N. A comparative investigation of the predictive validity of admissions criteria for Anglos, Blacks, and Mexican

Americans. Unpublished Ph.D. dissertation, The University of Texas at Austin, 1977.

Ekstrom, R. B. Issues of test bias and validity. Paper presented at the annual meeting of the American Psychological Association, New York, September 1979.

Evans, F. R., & Reilly, R. R. A study of speededness as a source of test bias. Journal of Educational Measurement, 1972, 9, 123-31.

Evans, F. R., & Reilly, R. A study of test speededness as a potential source of bias in the quantitative score of the Admission Test for Graduate Study in Business. Research in Higher Education, 1973, 1, 173-83.

Flaugher, R. L. Testing practices, minority groups, and higher education: A review and discussion of the research. Research Bulletin 70-41. Princeton, N.J.: Educational Testing Service, 1970.

French, J. W., & Dear, R. E. Effect of coaching on an aptitude test. Educational and Psychological Measurement, 1959, 19, 319-30.

García, J. Intelligence testing: quotients, quotes, and quackery. In J. L. Martínez, Jr. (Ed.), Chicano Psychology. New York: Academic Press, 1977, pp. 197-212.

Gheselli, E. E. Theory of psychological measurement. New York: McGraw-Hill, 1964.

Glenn, P. Anxiety and ethnicity of fourth-grade children. Unpublished Master's thesis, The University of Texas at Austin, 1969.

Goldman, L. Using tests in counseling (2nd ed.). New York: Appleton-Century-Crofts, 1971.

Goldman, R. D. Hidden opportunities in the prediction of college grades for different subgroups. Journal of Educational Measurement, 1973, 10, 205-10.

Goldman, R. D., & Hewitt, B. N. Predicting the success of Black, Chicano, Oriental, and White college students. Journal of Educational Measurement, 1976, 13, 107-18.

Goldman, R. D., & Richards, R. The SAT prediction of grades for Mexican American versus Anglo American students at the University of California, Riverside. Journal of Educational Measurement, 1974, 11, 129-35.

Hall, E. R. Motivation and achievement in Black and White junior college students. Journal of Social Psychology, 1975, 97, 107-13.

Hill, K. T. Anxiety in the evaluative context. Young Children, 1971, 27, 97-116.

Jacobson, R. L. Black enrollment rising sharply, U.S. data show. The Chronicle of Higher Education, October 4, 1971.

Kallingal, A. The prediction of grades of black and white students at Michigan State University. Journal of Educational Measurement, 1971, 8, 263-65.

Khan, S. B. The relative magnitude of speed and power in the SCAT. Journal of Educational Measurement, 1968, 5, 327-29.

Kirkland, M. C. The effects of tests on students and schools. Review of Educational Research, 1971, 41, 303-50.

Klineberg, O. Race differences. New York: Harper, 1935.

Lowman, R. P., & Spuck, D. W. Predictors of college success for the disadvantaged Mexican American. Journal of College Student Personnel, 1975, 16, 40-48.

Mercer, J. R. Pluralistic diagnosis in the evaluation of Black and Chicano children: A procedure for taking sociocultural variables into account in clinical assessment. In C. A. Hernandez, M. J. Haug, & N. N. Wagner (Eds.), Chicanos: Social and psychological perspectives. St. Louis: C. V. Mosby, 1976.

McClelland, D. C. Testing for competence rather than for "intelligence." American Psychologist, January 1973, 1-14.

National Board on Graduate Education. Minority group participation in graduate education. No. 5, June 1976.

Nieves, L. The GRE and the minority student: A perspective. Paper presented at the annual meeting of the American Psychological Association, Washington, D.C., September 1976.

Oliveira, A., Cárdenas, I., Cardoza, R., Carter, T., Muñoz, L. Rivera, F., Sánchez, W., & Valencia, A. Access to college for Mexican Americans in the southwest. College Entrance Examination Board, Higher Education Surveys, Report #6, 1972.

Olmedo, E. L. Psychological testing and the Chicano: A reassessment. In J. L. Martinez, Jr. (Ed.), Chicano Psychology. New York: Academic Press, 1977, pp. 175-95.

Padilla, A. M., & Ruiz, R. A. Latino mental health: A review of the literature. Washington, D.C.: U.S. Government Printing Office, 1973.

Peterson, J., Lanier, L. H., & White, H. M. Comparisons of white and negro children in certain ingenuity and speed tests. Journal of Comparative Psychology, 1925, 5, 271-83.

Pfeifer, C. M., & Sedlacek, W. E. The validity of academic predictors for black and white students at a predominantly white university. Journal of Educational Measurement, 1971, 8, 253-61.

Phillips, B. N. An analysis of causes of anxiety among children in school (Final Rep., Proj. No. 2616, U.S.O.E. Cooperative Research Branch). Austin, Tex.: University of Texas, 1966.

Phillips, B. N., Martin, R. P., & Meyers, J. School-related interventions with anxious children. In C. D. Spielberger (Ed.), Anxiety: Current trends in theory and research, Vol. 2. New York: Academic Press, 1972.

Pike, L. W. Short-term instruction, testwiseness, and the Scholastic Aptitude Test: A literature review with research recommendations. Research Bulletin 78-2. Princeton, N.J.: Educational Testing Service, 1978.

Pike, L. W., & Flaugher, R. L. Assessing the meaningfulness of group responses to multiple-choice test items. Reprinted from the Proceedings, 87th Annual Convention, American Psychological Association, 1970.

Poston, D. L., Jr., & Alvirez, D. On the cost of being a Mexican American worker. In Chicanos: Social and psychological perspectives. St. Louis: C. V. Mosby, 1976.

Reilly, R. R., & Evans, F. R. The effects of test time limits on the performance of culturally defined groups. Paper presented at the annual meeting of the American Educational Research Association, New Orleans, September 1974.

Rincón, E. T. Test speededness, test anxiety, and test perform- ance: A comparison of Mexican American and Anglo American high school juniors. Unpublished Ph.D. dissertation, The University of Texas at Austin, 1979.

Roberts, A. H., & Greene, J. E. Cross-cultural study of relationships among four dimensions of time perspective. Perceptual and Motor Skills, 1971, 33, 163-73.

Ruebuch, B. K. Anxiety. In H. W. Stevenson (Ed.), Sixty- second yearbook of the National Society for the Study of Education, part I, child psychology. Chicago: University of Chicago Press, 1963.

Samuda, R. J. Psychological testing of American minorities: Issues and consequences. New York: Harper & Row, 1975.

Sarason, I. G. Empirical findings and theoretical problems in the use of anxiety scales. Psychological Bulletin, 1960, 57, 403-15.

Schacter, S. The psychology of affiliation. Palo Alto, Calif.: Stanford University Press, 1969.

Shannon, L. Age change in time perception in Native Americans, Mexican Americans, and Anglo Americans. Journal of Cross- Cultural Psychology, 1976, 7, 117-22.

Slakter, M. J. Generality of risk taking on objective examinations. Educational and Psychological Measurement, 1969, 29, 115-28.

Slakter, M. J. The penalty for not guessing. Journal of Educa- tional Measurement, 1968(a), 5, 141-44.

Slakter, M. J. The effect of guessing strategy on objective test scores. Journal of Educational Measurement, 1968(b), 5, 217-29.

Spiegelberger, C. C. The effects of manifest anxiety on the academic achievement of college students. Mental Hygiene, 1962, 46, 420-26.

Stanley, J. C., & Porter, A. C. Correlation of Scholastic Aptitude Test scores with college grades for Negroes versus Whites. Journal of Educational Measurement, 1967, 4, 199-218

Swineford, F. Technical manual for users of test analysis. Statistical Report 56-42. Princeton, N.J.: Educational Testing Service, 1956.

Temp, G. Validity of the SAT for blacks and whites in thirteen integrated institutions. Journal of Educational Measurement, 1971, 8, 245-51.

Tseng, M. S., & Thompson, D. L. Need achievement, fear of failure, perception of occupational prestige, and occupational aspirations of adolescents of different socio-economic groups. Paper presented at the annual meeting of the American Educational Research Association, Los Angeles, February 1969.

U.S. Commission on Civil Rights. Mexican-American education study, Report II. The unfinished education: Outcomes for Minorities in the five southwestern states. Washington, D.C.: U.S. Government Printing Office, 1971.

Willingham, W. W. Predicting success in graduate education. A paper presented at the Graduate Record Examination Board's Research Seminar at the 12th annual meeting of the Council of Graduate Schools. Princeton, N.J.: Educational Testing Service, 1973.

Wine, J. Test anxiety and the direction of attention. Psychological Bulletin, 1971, 76, 92-104.

Wing, C. W., Jr., & Wallach, M. A. College admissions and the psychology of talent. New York: Holt, Rinehart & Winston, 1971.

Wrightstone, J. W. Relation of testing programs to teaching and learning. The impact and improvement of school testing programs. In W. G. Findley (Ed.), the Sixty-second yearbook of the National Society for the Study of Education, Part II. Chicago: University of Chicago Press, 1963, pp. 45-61.

6

ADMISSION OF CHICANO STUDENTS TO HIGHER EDUCATION: MODELS AND METHODS

Jude Valdez

The process of selecting minority students for college study has been subject to a great deal of criticism over the last several years (for example, Howard, 1968; Campbell, 1971; Crossland, 1971; Huber, 1971; Marston, 1971; Mares, 1973; Leslie & Gunne, 1973; Willingham, 1974; Fincher, 1975; Sedlacek & Brooks, 1976; Valdez, 1976; Breland, 1978). This criticism has generally focused on the employment of selection criteria poorly related to success in college, or the capriciousness of the selection process itself.

There is widespread opinion among educators that a reform, or modification, of the traditional admission process is long over-due. Two factors have provided a strong impetus for this. First, college educators are recognizing that successful completion of a degree program is a function of many factors—both academic and nonacademic (Heiss, 1970; Lenning et al., 1974). Indeed, university catalogs and higher education literature in general describe college education in terms of multiple objectives and, consequently, multiple success criteria. It seems reasonable then to expect that Chicano student selection should be based on multiple criteria related to the varied dimensions of success. A second imperative for change in the admissions process stems from the high attrition rates that are so common among minority students (Astin, 1975; Sedlacek & Brooks, 1976; Fetters, 1977; Noel, 1978; Pantages & Creedon, 1978). Attrition rates are sub-ject to several interpretations; but inasmuch as attrition reflects loss of resources and mismatch of students and programs, it is important to improve the selection process.

The traditional admission model in U.S. colleges and univer-sities has utilized grade-point averages and scores on standardized admission tests as determinants of selection. The shortcomings of this model lie in the almost exclusive use of these two selection criteria. Nonacademic dimensions of performance are rarely considered in any systematic fashion (Lenning et al., 1974; Fincher, 1975; Sedlacek & Brooks, 1976). Further, as Willingham (1974) points out, there are many important intellectual abilities not represented among the traditional selection measures, for example creativity, independent scholarship, rigorous thinking.

In response to criticisms of traditional admission methods, and to ensure that talented and deserving individuals are not automatically ruled out by failure to meet the traditional criteria, some colleges have begun to experiment with alternate admissions methods. These admissions have been variously designated as "provisional," "conditional," or "special." Typically, these admission programs have been used almost exclusively for minority students (Mares, 1973; Hamilton, 1973). The unfortunate result of this well-intentioned effort is that often minority status is equated with academic marginality.

Minority admission programs operate basically by waiving or adjusting traditional admission requirements, and then by attempting to gauge the applicant's potential for college work through some other means, usually letters of recommendation or personal interviews. The minority admission model reflects an attempt to ameliorate the perceived shortcomings of traditional admission practices by broadening selection criteria. However, the employment of this alternate model remains limited to certain exceptional situations. The call for reform in the minority admission process is broader than the development of an alternate strategy. It is a call for basic reform of the admission process through the development of selection criteria congruent with the multiple goals of college education. MacKinnon (1968), for instance, argues that admission officers should:

> . . . supplement intelligence and aptitude tests with independent measures of extracurricular achievement and originality, and if additional checks are to be used, with tests that tap those traits and motivational dispositions which have been shown to be positively related to creative striving and creative achievements. (p. 108)

The Educational Testing Service, one of the largest developers of standardized admission tests in the United States, repeatedly has cautioned those who make admission decisions that test scores are one element in a total picture and should be considered along with other data—not as a sole criterion for admission. Willingham (1974) makes a most convincing case for the development of more relevant selection strategies. He concludes:

> The best way to improve selection of . . . students
> will be to develop improved criteria for success.
> This is no small job for faculties, but it carries the
> promise of more effective utilization of talent and
> greater assurance of equity in admitting students
> to advanced training and the privilege associated
> with such training. (p. 278)

Although the use of multiple selection criteria is broadly endorsed, the development of administratively practical methods for identifying relevant selection criteria has yet to emerge.

PROBLEMS WITH ACADEMIC PREDICTION

The major focus of research dealing with admission of Chicanos to college has been on investigating traditional admission practices (Lavin, 1965; Lannholm, 1972; Willingham, 1974; Breland, 1978). Specifically, researchers have sought to assess the ability of test scores and/or grades from previous academic work to accurately predict success in college. Success has usually been defined in terms of grade-point averages in college work or completion of the degree program. The result of this research has been mixed and controversial. This controversy has developed primarily because of the tendency of minority students to score below their majority counterparts on predictive measures such as standardized admission tests (Coleman, 1966; Astin, 1970; Crossland, 1971; Stanley, 1971; Linn, 1973; Mayhew & Ford, 1974; Sedlacek & Brooks, 1976; Breland, 1978). The question of whether standardized predictors accurately estimate the academic potential of minority applicants (i.e., Chicanos) without bias remains unanswered.

The basic question is whether norm referenced admission instruments predict academic performance for Chicanos in the same way they do for the majority groups on whom the norms are based. The issue as pointed out above is not yet settled and the literature remains divided.

PROPOSALS FOR ALTERNATE ADMISSIONS SYSTEMS

Dissatisfaction with traditional college admission procedures has resulted in some proposals for alternate admission models that promise to be more sensitive to minority applicants. Houston and Roscoe (1968) have proposed the use of the judgment analysis technique in the selection of students for college work. This admission model calls for each college to define those abilities that characterize successful students. In considering a number of applicants for a position, each applicant is judged in relation to the criteria of success, and then measured against other applicants to arrive at a decision.

Koen (1969) has suggested that one way of developing more relevant selection criteria would be to have faculty identify those student qualities or attributes associated with successful college work. Additionally, useful information could be obtained by having students themselves participate in this process. Once these student qualities or attributes have been proposed, the next step is to attach weights of importance or significance to each of them. A list of attributes ranked in order of perceived functional importance would thus emerge. The list could then serve as a basis for a rating scale with which to judge prospective students.

Willingham (1974) has proposed the development of an alternate admission model based on multiple predictor and success variables related to academic program objectives. His model calls for a redefinition of success in terms of educational program objectives (for example, academic competence, teaching skills, involvement in professional affairs, innovative work, and so forth), and the identification of appropriate predictors of that success (for example, ability tests, grades, background characteristics, interests, and so forth). Willingham suggests that using variables of this sort for the selection and assessment of college students has the desirable effect of broadening the conception of success and talent.

Cole (1972), in discussing the effects of traditional admission criteria on minority students, has proposed an equal opportunity admission model to deal with measurement bias that may be intervening in the selection of minorities for higher education. She does not discount the use of tests or other predictors in the selection process, but suggests the development of more sensitive tests or predictors. This model places the burden of improving prediction on the selecting institution and even allows for different predictors for different groups. Under this model, the selecting institution and the potentially successful applicant both benefit from the use of tests and other predictors.

Sedlacek and Brooks (1976), in reviewing studies of nontraditional predictors useful in predicting minority student success in college, have identified seven key noncognitive variables. Among these seven variables are a positive self-concept, a realistic self-appraisal, the preference for long-range goals over short-term or immediate needs, availability of a strong support person, successful leadership experience, an ability to deal with racism, and demonstrated community service. The authors conclude that these variables can be practically assessed by counselors, through interviews, standardized measures, questionnaires, or application forms. The underlying goal of this alternate approach to minority admission is to collect the most useful information possible for making admission decisions. Ultimately, the authors state, utilization of this information on all applicants should result in an unbiased selection of students and an increase in minority students.

EXPERIMENTS WITH ALTERNATE ADMISSIONS

Leslie and Gunne (1973) conducted an assessment of 99 specially admitted and 115 regularly admitted students at Pennsylvania State University enrolled during the summer and fall terms of 1970. Regularly admitted students were those who met a universitywide requirement of 2.5 minimum grade-point average or the particular standards of the various departments of the university. Specially admitted students did not meet this requirement, but were considered potentially able in the judgment of admission officers. Faculty ratings of student performance were the success criteria used. The data analysis consisted of a factor analysis of the faculty ratings (on 11 items of a questionnaire) and analysis of variance of group mean factor scores.

The authors reported that essentially there were very few differences between specially admitted students and regularly admitted students when compared on a universitywide basis. There were only a few differences on comparisons within colleges. In short, "specially admitted students did not appear to differ importantly from (regular) traditional students in the perception of faculty members" (p. 98). A follow-up study found no significant differences in grade-point averages and in completion rates between both groups.

Carlisle (1968), in a paper prepared for the annual meeting of the Council of Graduate Schools, reported on a special minority graduate admission program at the University of California at Los Angeles. After several problems with initial cycles of the program, a modified version was implemented in 1966. The modification included increased financial support, improved advising and orientation as well as improved selection criteria utilizing, among other factors, undergraduate faculty recommendations. Carlisle reports that of 21 minority students admitted only one failed academically. In earlier versions of the program, nearly 25 percent of the students did not make satisfactory progress and had to withdraw. It is interesting to note, however, that a comparison of students who persisted with those who did not reveals that entering undergraduate grade-point averages did not appear to be a critical factor in success, at least within reasonable limits and assuming that other selection factors were taken into account.

In a paper delivered before the American College Personnel Association, Davis and Welty (1970) reported on an alternate admissions system used to select minority undergraduate students at Oberlin College. The objective at Oberlin was to develop admission criteria with which to select Black undergraduate students who had the greatest chance of succeeding in a college environment that was socially and culturally foreign to them. The enabling characteristic was termed "hipness" and consisted of competitiveness, high motivation, and self-reliance.

Three groups of Black students were admitted: 18 were not "hip" but met regular Oberlin admission criteria; 14 were both "hip" and met regular criteria; and seven were "hip" but did not meet regular criteria. At the end of the first semester, there was no appreciable difference in grade-point averages among the groups. Although the report presents summary impressions, the implications of motivation, competitiveness, and self-reliance on admissions at the undergraduate level indicate sufficient promise to warrant further investigation.

Valdez (1976) has developed and pilot tested a performance-centered model for identifying a comprehensive set of graduate student selection criteria at the departmental level. The significance of the study was that it demonstrated that viable strategies and methods exist for implementing minority-sensitive admission systems.

The model tested was an adaptation and expansion of the critical incident technique. A basic assumption of the study was that improved selection of students—both minority and nonminority—would emerge if the determinants of academic success could be identified. Once these determinants have been identified and empirically validated, then focus could be shifted toward employing them in admission programs.

Approximately 670 critical incidents, specific illustrations of most and least successful student performances, were collected from faculty and students in three participating departments of a major university. A taxonomy of 24 performance categories for sorting the incidents was developed by a team of faculty and student judges. To test the fit between the incidents and the performance categories of the taxonomy, a second group of judges sorted the incidents into performance categories. The 24 performance categories were then converted into rating scales with operationally defined poles.

The resulting instrument was the Student Performance Rating Scale (SPRS), which was used by faculty to rate a sample of currently enrolled students. A factor analysis of the ratings generated four broad and independent factors: Scholarship, Interpersonal Relationships, Stamina and Drive, and Leadership. The Scholarship factor included a complex of student performances associated with academic achievement. The Interpersonal Relationship factor described a student's interaction with others coupled with an ability to learn from them and contribute to their learning as well. The Stamina and Drive factor included the SPRS items that describe students' abilities to cope with their environment and direct their progress toward certain goals. Leadership, the final factor, included those SPRS items that place the student in circumstances where he or she can influence others.

Multiple regression analysis was employed to determine empirically the relationships of the four factors to successful performance. Independent faculty ratings of each student's overall performance were used as the dependent variable in the regression equation. Finally, to assist in interpreting the four SPRS factors, bivariate correlation and regression analysis between the four factors and selected admission, performance, and biographical variables were undertaken. A schematic representation of the model developed and pilot tested is presented in Figure 6.1.

Judging from the results achieved, the admissions model pilot tested represents a viable methodology for formulating a comprehensive set of admission criteria congruent with the needs of a particular college or university. Results revealed that the four factors together account for about 80 percent of what faculty members view as successful performance in the departments studied. While academic performance clearly was identified as a key to success in college, there were some significant non-academic performances as well (Interpersonal Relationships, Stamina and Drive, and Leadership). The findings also suggest the traditional selection methods based on entrance grade-point averages and standardized admission tests do not assess many of those skills necessary to succeed in the college in which the model was pilot tested. Finally, the model demonstrated that methodologies do exist that can improve the selection of college students, both minority and nonminority.

FIGURE 6.1

A Performance-Centered Model for Developing a Comprehensive Set of Admission Criteria

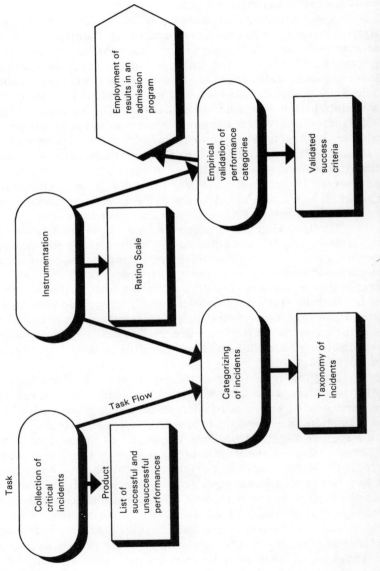

Source: Compiled by the authors

CONCLUSION

A great deal of criticism has been aimed at traditional admission practices in U.S. colleges and universities as they apply to minority students. This criticism has centered principally on the utilization of selection criteria poorly related to success. Educators have long recognized that success among college students is a function of many factors, academic as well as non-academic. Many researchers and college faculty have proposed the expansion of the present or traditional methods of admission to include a more comprehensive battery of selection criteria reflective of what in fact constitutes a successful performance in college. While this proposal has received broad endorsement, its implementation has been limited (Harvey, 1971; Mayhew & Ford, 1974; Willingham, 1974; Fincher, 1975).

One can draw several conclusions from the literature that is available on the admissions process:

1. The ability to predict which minority students will succeed in college based on traditional admission criteria is no better than modest.

2. Dissatisfaction with low correlations between standard selection and performance criteria has generated strong criticism of traditional admission practices, and has led some colleges to experiment with alternate admission systems.

3. Alternate admission systems, while holding some promise for equal educational opportunity, are but a temporary solution to the "admission problem."

4. Researchers and educators generally agree that better admission strategies will emerge as more comprehensive definitions of success in college are developed.

5. The need for effective methods of predicting minority student performance in college is critical.

REFERENCES

Astin, A. W. Preventing students from dropping out. San Francisco: Jossey-Bass, 1975.

Astin, A. W. Racial consideration in admission. In D. C. Nichols & O. Mills (Eds.), The campus and the racial crisis. Washington, D.C.: The American Council on Education, 1970.

Breland, H. M. Population validity and college entrance measures. Princeton, N.J.: Educational Testing Service, 1978.

Campbell, D. D. Admissions Policies: Side effects and their Implication. American Psychologist, 1971, 26, 636-48.

Carlisle, D. The disadvantaged student in graduate school masters and doctoral degree programs in predominantly non-Negro universities. Paper presented at the Eighth Annual Meeting of the Council of Graduate Schools in the U.S., December 1968.

Cole, N. Bias in selection. ACT Research Report Number 51. Iowa City, Iowa: ACT Publications, 1972.

Coleman, J. S. Equality of educational opportunity. Washington D.C.: U.S. Government Printing Office, 1966.

Crossland, F. E. Minority access to college. New York: Schock Books, 1971.

Davis, W. G., & Welty, G. A. The old systems and the new college students. Paper presented at the American College Personnel Association Convention, St. Louis, March 1970.

Fetters, W. B. Withdrawal from institutions of higher education: An appraisal with longitudinal data involving diverse institutions. Washington, D.C.: U.S. Government Printing Office, 1977.

Fincher, C. Strategies and trends in admission research. College and University, 1975, 51, 27-37.

Hamilton, I. B. Graduate school programs for minority/ disadvantaged students. Princeton, N.J.: Educational Testir Service, 1973.

Harvey, J. Graduate School Admissions. College and Universit Bulletin, November 1971, 4-5.

Heiss, A. Challenges to graduate schools. San Francisco: Jossey-Bass, 1970.

Houston, S., & Roscoe, J. The use of the judgement analysis technique in predicting success in graduate education. Washington, D.C.: American Personnel and Guidance Associa tion, 1968.

Howard, L. C. Graduate education for the "disadvantaged"
and Black-oriented university graduates. Washington, D.C.:
Council of Graduate Schools in the United States, 1968.

Huber, W. H. Channeling Students for Greater Retention.
College and University, 1971, 47, 19-29.

Koen, F. M. What are your objectives: Some implications for
admitting graduate students, training college teachers and
evaluating teaching. Paper presented at the Second Summer
Workshop for Graduate Deans, Lake Arrowhead, Calif.,
July 1969.

Lannholm, G. Summaries of GRE validity studies: 1966-1970.
Princeton, N.J.: Educational Testing Service, 1972.

Lavin, D. Prediction of academic performance. New York:
Russell Sage Foundation, 1965.

Lenning, O. T., Munday, L. A., Johnson, O. B., Vander Well,
A. R., & Brue, E. J. The many faces of college success
and their nonintellective correlates. Iowa City, Iowa: ACT
Publications, 1974.

Leslie, L., & Gunne, M. Success among specially admitted
graduate students. Education and Urban Society, 1973, 6,
85-101.

Linn, R. L. Fair test use in selection. Review of Educational
Research, 1973, 43, 139-61.

MacKinnon, D. Selecting students with creative potential. In
Heist (Ed.), The creative college student: An unmet challenge.
San Francisco: Jossey-Bass, 1968.

Mares, K. An investigation of differences perceived by adminis-
trators concerning critical factors related to programs for
the disadvantaged student in different types of higher education institutions. Unpublished Ph.D. thesis. University of
Missouri, Kansas City, 1973.

Marston, A. R. It is time to reconsider the Graduate Records
Examination. American Psychologist, 1971, 26, 653-56.

Mayhew, L., & Ford, P. Reform in graduate and professional
education. San Francisco: Jossey-Bass, 1974.

Noel, L. (Ed.). Reducing the dropout rate. San Francisco: Jossey-Bass, 1978.

Pantages, T. J., & Creedon, C. F. Studies of college attrition: 1950-1975. Review of Educational Research, 1978, 48, 49-101.

Sedlacek, W. E., & Brooks, G. C., Jr. Racism in American education: A model for change. Chicago: Nelson-Hall, 1976.

Stanley, J. C. Predicting college success of the educationally disadvantaged. Science, 1971, 171, 640-47.

Valdez, J. A Performance-centered model for generating graduate student selection criteria at the departmental level: An exploratory study. Unpublished Ph.D. dissertation, University of Texas at Austin, 1976.

Willingham, W. Predicting success in graduate education. Science, 1974, 183, 273-78.

7

A COMPARISON OF MINORITY STUDENTS' CONCERNS AT TWO UNIVERSITY CAMPUSES

Augustine Barón, Jr.,
Melba J. T. Vásquez, and Jude Valdez

With an ever increasing number of minority students enroll-
ing in college, student service personnel have begun focusing
attention on the needs of this growing population. In an effort
to begin the development of a data base for the development of
minority student services, needs assessments were conducted
first at the University of Texas in Austin (UT, Austin) and
then at Colorado State University (CSU) in Fort Collins. The
unique feature of these surveys is that the instrument used
was essentially the same, except for wording that was changed
to conform to each university environment. Thus, responses
from students can be directly compared so that differences between institutions can be deciphered.

The two universities are sufficiently different in size and
overall character. UT is one of the largest state universities
in the country with an enrollment of over 45,000 students. It
is located in a large city of 350,000 people that serves as the
capital of the state. CSU is located in a rural setting with a
population of about 80,000. Enrollment is currently set at 18,000.

OVERVIEW

Needs assessment for college populations has taken many
forms in recent years. Some strategies rely on the notion of
"person-environment fit" and consequently make use of standardized data collection instruments. Among these are the Activities
Index-College Characteristics Index (Stern, 1970), the College
and University Environment Scales (Pace, 1962) and the University Residence Environment Scale (Moos & Gerst, 1974). The
goal of such instruments is to assess the psychosocial environment
of the campus and to see if it matches the needs or desires of
the students.

Another approach is the eco-mapping system outlined by Aulepp and Delworth (1975). This approach has "person-environment fit" as part of its strategy; but it also attempts to assess the visibility and utilization patterns of various campus services and to compare these against expressed areas of student needs.

It is this second approach that was taken by the project reported in this article. Although the research did not make use of standard psychosocial environmental assessment instruments, many of the items included in the questionnaire employed in the project can be said to fall in the "ecological" category.

Recognizing the need for a comprehensive descriptive study of the University of Texas at Austin minority undergraduat population, the Research and Evaluation unit of the Dean of Students Office early in the 1977 Spring semester began to explor the possibility of undertaking such a study. Meetings and consultations were held with faculty, campus services staff, individu students, and student groups. The Minority Student Services Unit of the Dean of Students Office served as the facilitator for the meetings. These discussions were critical in focusing the need and rationale for a study of minority undergraduate student A consensus gradually emerged that a comprehensive study of minority students should have several purposes, including the following: first, a description of the population in terms of demographic characteristics; second, an assessment of student needs and concerns; third, a survey of primary communicational networks, places of residence, sources of financial and personal support, and extracurricular activities; and fourth, an analysis of the visibility and utilization of campus services. This present report focuses on all but the last of these findings.

An initial survey focusing on Chicano and Black UT student was conducted during the Spring semester of 1977. A second survey that incorporated Anglo, Black, and Chicano students was carried out during the Fall semester of 1977. This report is based on data collected from both surveys.

The UT, Austin Sample

A random sample of students at UT was drawn that consisted of Anglo, Black, and Chicano undergraduates who were enrolled as of the twelfth class day of the Fall 1977 semester. The sample contained 1,273 individuals stratified by sex and classification within ethnicity, and included 697 Anglo students (366 men and 331 women), 236 Black students (94 men and 142 women), and 340 Chicano students (197 men and 143 women). Returned by the sample were 1,304 questionnaires. However, only 1,273 were usable, resulting in an overall response rate of 64 percent.

The CSU Sample

A random sample of students was drawn from lists of Anglo, Black, Chicano, Asian, and Native American undergraduates who were enrolled in the Spring 1979 semester. Usable questionnaires numbering 442 were returned resulting in an overall response rate of 49 percent. Since much of the data is reported by ethnicity, it is important to note the representation of each ethnic group. The sample included 182 Anglo students (106 males, 76 females), which comprised 1 percent of the Anglo population at CSU in the Spring of 1979; 47 Black students (16 males, 31 females), 31 percent of the Black population; 105 Chicano students (56 males, 49 females), 35 percent of the Chicano student population; 82 Asian-American students (34 males, 47 females), 47 percent of the Asian-American student population; 14 Native American students (12 males, 2 females), 30 percent of the Native American student population, and 8 "other" students. There were 26 of the Chicano students (15 males and 11 female) who chose to identify themselves as other than "Chicano" or "Mexican-American," for example, "Spanish-American," American of Spanish descent, and so forth. Because of some hypotheses that different ways of identifying oneself in the Hispanic population is associated with different ideologies and outlooks, separate analyses were performed for these two groups throughout the investigation. Thus, there were two Hispanic groups: 79 Chicano students (42 males, 37 females) and 26 "other Hispanic students" (15 male and 11 female). Data from the CSU survey presented here will concentrate on Anglo, Black, Chicano, and "other Hispanic" groups.

Data Collection Instrument

Working in concert with selected faculty, staff, students, and student peer counselors, the UT Research and Evaluation Unit developed a survey instrument that was pilot tested with a group of 40 minority students. The product that emerged was the "Student Needs Survey." Several features of the instrument are noteworthy: first, the instrument was designed to be completed in about 20 minutes; second, an identifying number on each instrument allowed the data to be linked to the university's student data base, which in turn permitted access to the students' academic records and demographic files; third, several open-ended questions at the end of the instrument provided the respondents a forum to comment freely on a variety of issues. A cover letter to the questionnaire was prepared explaining the purpose of the study and assuring the student of confidentiality.

The survey instrument consisted of three sections. In the first section students rated 63 items on a five-point Likert-type scale according to the amount of concern elicited by the item. A response of "1" indicated that the item was not a problem, while a response of "2" indicated the item was a minor problem; a "3" indicated a moderate problem; "4" a major problem; and a response of "5" designated the item as a crisis. These multiple-choice questions represented six areas of student concern: Academic concerns (19 items), Minority concerns (11 items), Financial concerns (10 items), Environmental concerns (7 items), Interpersonal concerns (11 items), and Career concerns (5 items). Questions regarding the students' needs, utilization, and knowledge of 17 campus agencies were asked in the second section. The third section was comprised of multiple-choice items for self-reported characteristics and open-ended questions asking students how they might change the university (Pitcher, 1978).

Basically the same instrument was used at CSU with modifications in wording made so as to make the survey compatible with terms used on that campus.

RESULTS

Place of Residence at UT

Based on the replies of the respondents to the survey, it was found that 50 percent of the Chicanos live off campus and 3 percent live in cooperative housing. About 47 percent of the Blacks live off campus, 45 percent live in residence halls, and 3 percent live in co-ops. By comparison, less than 8 percent of the total UT, Austin student population (mostly Anglos) live in university housing. Approximately 43 percent of Black and Chicano respondents reported living in such housing.

Place of Residence at CSU

Larger percentages of ethnic minority students live in residence halls than do Anglo students (38 percent to 49 percent compared to 32.4 percent). A large percentage of minority students may thus be exposed to an environment generally considered less conducive to studying. On the other hand, there is a "captured" group of students for special programs.

Personal Income at UT

Regarding personal annual income, 59 percent of the Chicano respondents indicated an income between $2,000 and $3,900 as opposed to 54 percent of the Blacks. Twenty-four percent of the Chicanos and 30 percent of the Blacks had less than $2,000 of income. Nine percent of the Chicanos and 12 percent of the Blacks had incomes between $4,000 and $5,900, and 8 percent of the Chicanos and 4 percent of the Blacks indicated an income of $6,000 or over. The majority of Anglos had incomes above $4,000. The University's Financial Aid Office estimated that for the academic year 1976-77, a student needed $3,200 to meet his or her educational expenses.

Personal Income at CSU

The CSU survey project included more specific analyses of personal income than did the UT project. This was done because the UT data indicated that personal finances were a major area of concern. Consequently, detailed information was obtained with the CSU survey to elaborate various facets of income, including an analysis of parental education and class level.
As expected, ethnic minorities' parental income at CSU was considerably lower than Anglos. The mean parental income for Anglo students was $20,000 to $24,000 while Black and Chicano students reported parental mean incomes of $15,000 to $19,999. The only exception to this profile was the "other Hispanic" group, whose parental income profile was very similar to that reported by Anglo students.
Astin (1975) concluded that receiving support from parents for college expenses generally enhances the student's ability to complete college (except for women from high income brackets). The extent to which financial aid and other student assistance programs have compensated for disparities in financial circumstances is unclear; but generally, Astin (1975) found scholarships or grants associated with small increases in student persistence rates. Participation in work study programs also appears to enhance student persistence. Reliance on savings, on the other

hand, decreases students' chances of finishing college as does
reliance on loans for men in all income groups. Effects of reliance
on loans for women is highly variable.

Interesting patterns of differences regarding financial
sources of education were found for the students at CSU. Student
were to identify whether a particular financial source was: a
major source; a minor source; or not a source at all.

Largest percentages of ethnic groups including Blacks
(59.6 percent), Chicanos (46.8 percent), and "other Hispanics"
(50.0 percent) listed scholarships or grants as their major source
of finances. Anglo students (60.5 percent) used parental aid
as their major source of finances. While personal savings was
not used by a large number of students as a major source,
approximately one-third of Anglos and Chicanos did report using
savings as a major source. Many others used savings as a minor
source. Almost half of the Chicano students (43.0 percent) used
employment as a major source while approximately one-third of
the Anglo and of the "other Hispanic" groups used employment
as a source. "Other Hispanic" students reported the largest
percentages using loans as a major source of finances (42.3
percent) while over one-third of Blacks and Chicanos (38.3
percent and 38.0 percent respectively) used loans as a major
source.

Generally, if Astin's (1975) findings bear out with CSU
students, it is gratifying that the largest percentages of all
groups receive finances from sources that enhance persistence.
Resources could perhaps be even better distributed given some
still large percentages of students using loans and savings.

Educational Background of CSU Students' Parents

For the most part, similar trends were found in regard to
father's and mother's education, with larger percentages of
minority students' parents at lower levels than Anglo students'
parents. There were some interesting exceptions: "other Hispanics" once again enjoyed a similar profile compared to Anglos.
Almost three-fourths of both groups' fathers had attended college
(73.0 percent and 70.3 percent respectively). Black students
reported that well over half of their fathers had attended colleges
(63.8 percent). Chicano students reported the lowest levels of
father education (41.0 percent respectively). One-fifth (20.3
percent) of Chicano fathers had only a grammar school education.

Black students reported the highest level of education
for mothers, (63.8 percent had attended college or graduated

from college), followed by Anglo (59.9 percent), and "other Hispanic" (46 percent) students' mothers. Chicano students once again emerge with lowest percentages of mothers' educational levels (21.5 percent had attended college or graduated from college). A large group of ethnic minority students are first-generation college students.

There were also differences in parents' occupations among the groups (levels of occupations measured by International Scale of Occupations, Manaster & Havighurst, 1972). Once again, Anglo and "other Hispanic" students had fathers in the highest levels compared to other groups (52.7 percent and 50 percent in the top two levels respectively). Black and Chicano parents reported fewest father occupations that fell in the top two levels (25.5 percent and 24.1 percent respectively) and highest percentages in the two lowest levels, semi-skilled and unskilled.

Differences were less clear among groups for mothers' occupational level, largely because many mothers were reported to be housewives. Black students reported highest percentages of mothers to be in the two highest occupational levels (21.3 percent) followed by Anglo (14.2 percent) students' mothers, with "other Hispanic" and Chicano students reporting the most similar figures on this index: only 11.5 percent and 10.1 percent of their mothers respectively had occupations in the top two levels. Interestingly, Black students reported fewest (14.9 percent) of their mothers to be housewives. This figure is in correspondence with the figure reporting that Black students had mothers with highest levels of education.

Support Person at UT

With regard to persons upon whom minority persons rely for help in solving a personal or academic problem, results indicate that 45 percent of the sample rely on their fellow students for such help with another 18 percent indicating they have no support person and 13 percent indicating they rely on a faculty member.

Support Person at CSU

The largest percentages of students for each ethnic group at CSU count on other students for their support (28.6 to 62.2 percent). Faculty members were the second most frequently chosen support person (14.3 to 24.2 percent). The "other" category included miscellaneous persons such as: relative, friend off campus, priest or minister. A few students did indicate "no one" to whom they could turn.

Membership in Student Organizations at UT

It was also found that approximately 50 percent of the Chicano and Black respondents belonged to at least one organization. This is in comparison to approximately 35 percent of the total UT, Austin population that belong to at least one student organization.

Membership in Student Organizations at CSU

While a large number of students (31.9 percent to 46.9 percent) do not belong to any organization, most students belong to at least one organization. In some cases, larger percentages of ethnic minority students (Black, Chicano, and "other Hispanic" students) are affiliated with some association compared to Anglo students. This hopefully reflects that needs for affiliation are being met to some degree for most students.

Primary Sources of Information at UT

Regarding primary sources of information about campus services, 61 percent of the respondents indicated that their information comes from other students, and 54 percent indicated that the school newspaper, the Daily Texas, provided them with such information. (Multiple responses were permitted to this question. Consequently, total percentages exceed 100 percent.) Twenty-six percent of the respondents indicated that posters were their primary source of information, and another 13 percent rely on new student orientation for information.

Primary Sources of Information at CSU

The great majority of students (53.2 percent to 72.1 percent) get their information primarily from other students. The next major source for most groups (11.5 to 17.1 percent) was The Journal, the student newspaper. Almost 20 percent of Black and Chicano students get their information primarily from

the respective special support services set up for each of those
two groups: Black Student Services and El Centro Chicano. But
"word of mouth" seems to continue to be the primary source of
information for students.

Students' Concerns at UT

Table 7.1 lists the top 15 concerns from the group of 63
multiple-choice items comprising the 6 categories included in the
survey. Percentages of students from each ethnic and sex subgroup indicating each item as a major problem or crisis are also
noted. Considerable variability was apparent across sex and
ethnicity in regard to the order and content of the top concerns.
Four items, however, were among the top 15 for all groups:
influencing the administration, finding a part-time job compatible
with school, postponing luxuries until graduation, and budgeting
finances over the academic year. Minority students shared
several concerns not reported by Anglo students: the number
of minority faculty and staff, high school preparation, debts
for education, ability to do well on exams, and deciding what to
study.
      Financial concern items accounted for several of the over-
all top student concerns. Of the top 15 student concerns, 27
percent were financial for Anglo women, 33 percent for Anglo
men and Black women, 10 percent for Chicano women, and 47
percent for Black and Chicano men.
      Academic concerns also accounted for a sizable number
of the top 15 concerns. Across all six subgroups, from 27 to
40 percent of the top concerns were academically related. Although no academic items appeared consistently across each
minority group, several were evident across each minority group.
Two of these three concerns were ability-related, emphasizing
the finding that minority students are more concerned than
Anglos about academic ability.

Students' Concerns at CSU

Table 7.2 lists the top 15 concerns as expressed by Anglo,
Black, and Chicano students in the CSU sample. As was the
case with the UT sample, considerable variability appeared across
sex and ethnicity in regard to the order and content of the top
concerns. Four items also emerged across all the groups (except
for the "other Hispanic" groups): finding an affordable place to

TABLE 7.1

Percentages of UT, Austin Students Reporting Most Highly Ranked Concerns as Major Problems or Crises

	Anglo				Black				Chicano			
	Men	%	Women	%	Men	%	Women	%	Men	%	Women	%
1.	Influence the administration	30*	Influence the administration	32*	Number of minority faculty & staff	50*	Number of minority faculty & staff	54*	Job compatible with school	38*	Job compatible with school	40*
2.	Part-time job compatible with school	27*	Inexpensive place to live	30	Number of minority students	35	Job compatible with school	47*	Influence administration	34*	Postponing luxuries	34*
3.	Inexpensive place to live	26	Job compatible with school	29*	Influence the administration	34*	Influence administration	44*	High school preparation	31+	Influence administration	33*
4.	Choosing a career	23	Finding job after graduation	26	Recognition of unique minority needs	32*	Number of minority students	40	Inexpensive place to live	29	Inexpensive place to live	28
5.	Admittance to graduate school	23	Choosing a career	25	High school preparation	30	Recognition of unique needs of minorities	37	Admittance to graduate school	28	Debts for education	28+
6.	Finding time to study	22	Impersonal treatment	24	Job compatible with school	29+	Budgeting finances for year	36*	Postponing luxuries	28*	Admittance to graduate school	28
7.	Course scheduling	22	Finding time to study	22	Budgeting finances for year	28	Postponing luxuries	36*	Debts for education	27*	Budgeting finances for year	28*
8.	Postponing luxuries	20*	Budgeting finances for year	21*	Ability to do well on exams	26*	Ability to do well on exams	30+	Ability to do well on exams	26+	Math and science course ability	26
9.	Inexpensive meals	20	Seeking academic advice	21	Spending education money for emergencies	25+	Debts for education	30+	Number of minority faculty & staff	24+	High school preparation	25+
10.	Budgeting finances for yr	19*	Deciding what to study	20	Deciding what to study	24	Admittance to graduate school	30	Deciding what to study	24*	Deciding what to study	25*
11.	Find job after graduation	18	Postponing luxuries	20*	Financial burden on parents	24+	Math & science course ability	29+	Math & science course ability	22	Ability to do well on exams	24+
12.	Impersonal treatment	16	Course scheduling	19	Debts for education	22	Deciding what to study	28	Using educational money for emergency	22	Find job after graduation	24
13.	Writing papers	16	Math & science course ability	19	Finding out about financial aid	22+	Financial burden on parents	28+	Finding inexpensive meals	21	Financial burden on parents	24
14.	Concentrating on assignments	15	Large class size	18	Getting outside course help	21	High school preparation	27	Budgeting finances for year	20*	Number of minority faculty & staff	23+
15.	Seeking academic advice	15	Writing papers	18	Finding job after graduation	21	Finding job after graduation	21	Finding job after graduation	20	Finding time to study	22

*Among top 15 concerns across all groups.

+Among top 15 concerns across minority groups.

Source: Gayle Pitcher, Survey Reports 1–6. Austin, Tex.: Dean of Students Office, University of Texas, 1978. Reprinted by permission.

TABLE 7.2

Percentages of CSU Students Reporting Most Highly Ranked
Concerns as Major Problems or Crises

	Anglo			
	Men	%	Women	%
1.	Influencing the administration	23.9*	Part-time job compatible with school	30.9*
2.	Affordable place to live	23.7	Postponing luxuries	26.8*
3.	Choosing a career	22.6	Inexpensive meals	26.4
4.	Part-time job compatible with school	20.7*	Finding library materials	24.9
5.	Large size of classes	17.9	Ability in math & science	22.6
6.	Availability of lab equipment	17.9	Financial burden on parents	22.2
7.	Postponing luxuries	16.5*	Budgeting finances for semester	22.2
8.	Debts for educational loans	16.1	Affordable place to live	21.7
9.	Finding library materials	14.6	Influencing the administration	21.5*
10.	Being admitted to professional or graduate school	14.1	Debts for educational loans	20.0
11.	High school preparation	13.6	High school preparation	19.7
12.	Impersonal treatment	13.5	Choosing a major	19.7
13.	Financial burden on parents	13.0	Availability of lab equipment	18.5
14.	Choosing a major	12.7	Uncertainty of present major	17.3
15.	Having to use money set aside for education	11.2	Finding out about financial aid	17.2

*Among top 15 concerns across all groups.
+Among top 15 concerns across all minority groups.
Source: Compiled by the authors.

131

Table 7.2 (continued)

	Black			
	Men	%	Women	%
1.	Pertinent cultural events in Fort Collins	43.8	Number of minority students at Colorado State University	48.4+
2.	Number of minority students at Colorado State University	43.8+	Number of minority GTAs, faculty, and staff	48.4+
3.	Debts for educational loans	43.8+	Part-time job compatible with school	46.4*
4.	Part-time job compatible with school	42.9*	Debts for educational loans	42.9+
5.	Affordable place to live	31.3*	Ability in math and science	36.7
6.	Postponing luxuries	26.7*	Affordable place to live	36.7*
7.	Having to use money set aside for emergencies	26.6	Budgeting finances for semester	33.3
8.	Number of minority teaching assistants, faculty, and staff	25.1+	Postponing luxuries	33.3*
9.	Finding out about financial aid	25.0	Pertinent cultural events in Fort Collins	32.2
10.	Transportation to campus	25.0	Influencing the administration	27.5*
11.	Influencing the administration	23.1*	Ability to do well on exams	22.6
12.	University recognition of minority needs	20.0	University recognition of minority needs	22.3
13.	Getting academic advising	20.0	Financial burden on on parents	22.2
14.	Inexpensive meals	20.0	Getting to know minorities in Fort Collins	21.5
15.	Financial burden on parents	20.0	Ability to do well academically at Colorado State University	21.4

	Chicano			
	Men	%	Women	%
1.	Postponing luxuries	37.0*	Postponing luxuries	26.7*
2.	Influencing the administration	30.7*	Finding library materials	25.5
3.	Part-time job compatible with school	27.5*	Part-time job compatible with school	18.9*
4.	Debts for educational loans	27.0+	Budgeting finances for semester	18.9
5.	Being admitted to professional or graduate school	20.6	Ability in math and science	18.9
6.	Affordable place to live	20.5*	Number of minority students at Colorado State University	18.9+
7.	Number of minority teaching assistants, faculty, and staff	20.0+	Number of minority GTAs, faculty, and staff	18.9+
8.	Finding out about financial aid	19.5	Learning about jobs after graduation	16.7
9.	Large size of classes	19.5	Uncertainty of present major	16.7
10.	Ability to do well in exams	19.5	University recognition of minority needs	16.7
11.	Asking questions in class	17.5	Debts for educational loans	14.3+
12.	Inexpensive meal	17.5	Financial burden on parents	13.9
13.	Number of minority students at Colorado State University	17.5+	High school preparation	13.5
14.	Finding library materials	17.5	Influencing the administration	12.2*
15.	Unfair treatment from landlords	16.6	Affordable place to live	11.8

live, postponing luxuries until graduation, finding a part-time job compatible with school, and influencing the administration. Concerns specific to all ethnic subgroups (except for "other Hispanics) included: the number of minority students at CSU, debts for education, and the number of minority faculty and staff.

As is the case with the UT sample, financial concerns emerged as a major cluster of concerns. However, academic concerns did not form a second group of consistently major concerns for the CSU sample.

DISCUSSION

Comparing results between both campuses underscores more similarities than differences. Places of residence are quite similar. Large percentages of students (especially minority students) live in university housing. Personal income characteristics are less directly comparable since the CSU survey conducted more extensive investigation of this area than did the UT project. As noted earlier, however, students at CSU appear to be receiving the kinds of financial support that are considered to enhance persistence in college (Astin, 1975).

Another similarity involves support persons relied upon by students at each campus. Fellow students are the primary sources of such support. Membership in student organizations can be a sign of levels of comfort and "belongingness" to the campus environment. Both surveys found significant numbers of minority students belonging to at least one organization. Primary sources of information are also quite similar for both schools. The school newspaper is one of the major modes for acquiring information.

Regarding students' concerns, there are commonalities and interesting differences. Financial concerns are shared by all students regardless of ethnicity or sex. However, UT minority students cite a number of academically related concerns that do not appear consistently in the CSU sample. UT students are more concerned that CSU students with their high school preparation, ability to do well on exams, and deciding on a major. Thus, the UT minority students have additional academic concerns that may well arise from the pressures of being at a large, competitive institution. Further research is warranted on institutional differences regarding the academic preparation of minority students entering each university and the level of academic demands placed on students by each school.

Perhaps the most interesting differences that emerge from this study especially as they relate to Chicano psychology are those pertaining to the "other Hispanic" group surveyed at CSU. As noted earlier, 26 students chose to identify themselves as other than Chicano or Mexican-American. Because differences in ways of identifying oneself within Hispanic cultures is hypothesized as being associated with differing ideologies, acculturational levels, and so forth (Vásquez, 1978), separate analyses were conducted throughout the study at CSU.

The "other Hispanic" group had parental incomes and educational backgrounds most similar to the Anglo sample. Anglo and "other Hispanic" students also had fathers at the highest occupational levels. Regarding their top 15 concerns, "other Hispanic" students shared only two concerns with the remaining subgroups: influencing the administration and finding a part-time job compatible with school. "Other Hispanic" males had one item that they shared with the other minority subgroups: the number of minority students at CSU. This item was not among the top 15 for "other Hispanic" females.

These differences indicate that "other Hispanic" students at CSU are sufficiently different from the other minority groups in terms of parents' economic and educational background and concerns as expressed in the survey. Such differences point to the importance of class and possible acculturational factors among some Hispanic students that need to be taken into account when planning special student services.

Overall, then, the twin surveys reported here provide a normative base from which to compare and contrast students' expressed concerns across other campuses. In addition, interesting variations within and across groups by sex and ethnicity point to future research endeavors. These include institutional differences in terms of academic preparation of entering students, academic demands, and acculturation/class differences among various minority subgroups.

REFERENCES

Astin, A. W. Preventing students from dropping out. San Francisco: Jossey-Bass, 1975.

Aulepp, L., & Delworth, U. A Training manual for an ecosystem model. Boulder, Co.: Western Interstate Commission for Higher Education, 1975.

Manaster, G. J., & Havighurst, P. I. Cross national research: social psychological methods and problems. Boston: Houghton Mifflin, 1972.

Moos, R., & Gerst, R. University residence environment scale manual. Palo Alto, Ca.: Consulting Psychologists Press, 1974.

Pace, C. R. CUES: College & university environment scales. Princeton, N.J.: Educational Testing Service, 1962.

Pitcher, G. Survey Reports 1-6. Austin, Tex.: Dean of Student Office, University of Texas, 1978.

Stern, G. G. People in context: Measuring person-environment congruence in education and industry. New York: Wiley, 1970.

Vásquez, M. J. Chicano and Anglo university women: Factors related to their performance, persistence and attrition. Unpublished Ph.D. dissertation, University of Texas at Austin, 1978.

PART III
MENTAL HEALTH: ISSUES AND RESEARCH

8

MEXICAN-AMERICAN USAGE OF MENTAL HEALTH FACILITIES: UNDERUTILIZATION CONSIDERED

Steven López

Past reviews of Mexican-American[1] utilization of mental health facilities, with the exception of Barrera (1978), have concluded that this minority group consistently underutilizes services (Acosta, 1977, 1979; Padilla & Ruiz, 1973; Padilla, Ruiz, & Álvarez, 1975). These reviews have served an important role in bringing national attention to the mental health needs of the Mexican-American community and in identifying critical issues in the delivery of services to this ethnic group. However, there is a growing number of recent studies and statistical reports that indicate Mexican-Americans are utilizing mental health services in parity with their representation in the community (e.g., Sánchez, Acosta, & Grosser, 1979; Treviño, Bruhn, & Bunce, 1979). Moreover, some studies conducted over ten years ago also did not consistently support the often-cited conclusion of

Preparation of this manuscript was supported in part by a research grant awarded to the author from the Institute of American Cultures and the Chicano Studies Research Center, University of California at Los Angeles, and in part by Research Grant MH 24854 from the National Institute of Mental Health to the Spanish Speaking Mental Health Research Center at the University of California at Los Angeles, Amado M. Padilla, Principal Investigator. Sincere appreciation is extended to Martha Bernal and René Ruiz for their helpful, critical comments on earlier drafts. The author also wishes to thank Nelba Chávez, Leticia Cuecuecha-López, Israel Cuéllar, Antonio López, Amado Padilla, and Josefina Veloz for their helpful comments. An earlier version of this work was presented at the Western Psychological Association Convention in San Diego, 1979.

underutilization (for example, Jaco, 1959, 1960; Libo, Dunbar, & Warren, 1962; Wignall & Koppin, 1967). Given these findings, it is necessary to reconsider the conclusion that Mexican-American underutilize mental health services. The purpose of this chapter is threefold: first, to critically reexamine the research literature in order to reassess Mexican-American usage of mental health services; second, to identify significant conceptual and methodological limitations in this research; and third, to offer recommendations for future research.

The chapter is organized into five sections. The definitions of utilization status (that is, underutilization) are reviewed and evaluated in the first section. The next section contains a comprehensive review of three decades of research. Next, methodological limitations are identified and recommendations to improve them are provided. In the fourth section, future directions in utilization research are considered. Finally, there is a discussion of the implications of the findings and recommendations.

DEFINITIONS OF UTILIZATION STATUS

In order to assess utilization status of Mexican-Americans or any group, a comparison has to be made between the utilization rate of the said group and some standard. The critical question becomes, what is the most significant comparison group or standard? In the utilization literature, the most frequently used method compared the percentage of Mexican-Americans in the patient population with their percentage in the community or catchment area. Underutilization is then defined as the patient percentage being lower than the community percentage. Correlational analyses are sometimes conducted with this approach (for example, Cuéllar, 1978). A second method compares the admissions rates of Mexican-Americans with that of Anglo-Americans. Admissions rates are calculated by dividing the number of admissions of a given ethnic group by the number of persons of that group in a given catchment area. This proportion is then multiplied by a population factor that varies from 1,000 to 100,000 persons. Underutilization is reported when the Mexican-American admissions rate is less than that of Anglo-Americans.

These methods are rather straightforward and utilization status can be easily assessed. However, neither method takes into consideration the most critical factor in assessing utilization status, namely, the need for mental health services. The first approach assumes that the need for services is directly proportional to that group's representation in the community. For example, if there are 25 percent Mexican-Americans in the community, then their need is assumed to result in 25 percent of all admissions. Both approaches are based on the assumption that the need for services is equivalent across all groups. This is most obvious in the second approach; any significant deviation from the Anglo admission rate is considered over- or underutilization. The fact that Mexican-Americans may have a greater need for psychological help is not taken into consideration. Conceivably, Mexican-Americans could be overutilizing services as compared to Anglos; yet, when compared to their need, they could very likely be underutilizing services.

Psychiatric epidemiological research comparing Mexican-Americans with other ethnic groups is far from conclusive (Roberts, 1980). However, significant differences between Mexican-Americans and other groups have been found for general indexes of psychological distress.[2] These findings suggest that in order to properly assess the utilization status of Mexican-Americans, it is necessary to incorporate measures of need with measures of utilization. The manner in which this can be done is addressed later in this chapter.

MEXICAN-AMERICAN UTILIZATION RESEARCH: A REVIEW

With few exceptions, utilization status has been assessed by comparing patient population and catchment area percentages. For this review, the percentage approach is used to describe the results whenever possible so that cross-study comparisons can be made. The readers are cautioned that the findings of this review, as well as past reviews, are based on this limited approach since need-based utilization research has yet to be conducted with Mexican-Americans.

The research reviewed below and in Table 8.1 is organized according to the decade in which the data were collected rather than when they were actually published; single versus multiple institution studies; and whenever possible, the types of institutions where data were collected (for example, inpatient versus outpatient). Empirical research, case studies, and statistical reports published before September 1980 serve as the basis for this review.[3] In addition, studies that contain pertinent utilization data are included even though the study of utilization may not have been their focus (for example, Heiman & Kahn, 1977).

TABLE 8.1

Mexican-American Mental Health Services Utilization Studies/Reports by Decade

Study/Report	Time Period	Facility Type	Community	Percentage of MAs[a] in Patient Population or MA Admission Rate	Percentage of MAs in Community or Admission Rate of Comparison Group	MA Utilization Status[b]
1950s Multiple Institutions						
Jaco (1959)[c]	1951-52	Public	Texas	31 per 100,000	32 per 100,000 Anglos	+
	1951-52	Private	Texas	11 per 100,000	48 per 100,000 Anglos	−
1950s Single Institution						
Libo, Dunbar, & Warren (1962)	1958-59	State Hospital	New Mexico	41.8%	36.4%	+
1960s Multiple Institutions						
Bloom (1975)[d]	1959-61	Public Inpatient	Pueblo County, Colorado	18.3%	21.5%	−
	1959-61	Private Inpatient	Pueblo County, Colorado	13.6%	21.5%	−
Karno & Edgerton (1969)	Fiscal Year 1962/63	State Hospitals	California	2.2%	9-10%	−
	Fiscal Year 1962/63	State Mental Health Clinics	California	3.4%	9-10%	−
	Fiscal Year 1962/63	State-Local Inpatient	California	2.3%	9-10%	−

Study	Dates	Institution	Location			
	Fiscal Year 1962/63	Neuropsychiatric Institute Outpatient Clinics	California	.9%	9-10%	−
	June 30, 1966	State Hospitals	California	3.3%	9-10%	−
1960s Single Institution Karno (1966)	January 1, 1958-April 30, 1962	NPI Outpatient Clinic	Los Angeles	.8%	9.5-10.5%	−
Wignall & Koppin (1967, Reference Note 4)	Fiscal Year 1960/61	State Hospital	34 counties of Colorado	13.29% or 2.54 per 1000 MAs	9.25% or 1.34 per 1000 non-MAs	+
Pokorny & Frazier (1966)	July 1, 1966	State Hospital	Texas	11.6%	14.8%	−
Karno & Morales (1971)	Summer 1967	County Out-patient Center	East Los Angeles	86%	Not mentioned	+e
Torrey (1972, Note 5)	1968	Community Mental Health Center (CMHC)	Santa Clara County, California	4%	10%	−
Philippus (1971)	September 1967-January 1970	Mental Health Team Services	Denver	70%, 35%, 50% to 65%	68%	−
1970s Multiple Institutions Bloom (1975)d	September 1, 1969-August 31, 1971	Public Inpatient	Pueblo County,	34%	31.4%	+

(continued)

Table 8.1 (continued)

Study/Report	Time Period	Facility Type	Community	Percentage of MAs[a] in Patient Population or MA Admission Rate	Percentage of MAs in Community or Admission Rate of Comparison Group	MA Utilization Status[b]
Los Angeles County (1973)	September 1, 1969–August 31, 1971	Private Inpatient	Pueblo County, Colorado	23.5%	31.4%	–
	July 1970–June 1971	Outpatient Clinics	Los Angeles County	10.3%	18.3%	–
	July 1970–June 1971	Inpatient	Los Angeles County	9.6%	18.3%	–
Sue (1977)	1971–73	17 CMHCs*	Greater Seattle area	.6%	1.8%	–
Kruger (1974)	Fiscal Year 1972	24 CMH/MR Centers	Texas catchment areas	19.5%	18.3%	+
	Fiscal Year 1972	State Hospitals	Texas	11.1%	12.5%	–
Los Angeles County (1975)	July 1973–June 1974	Outpatient Clinics	Los Angeles County	14.3%	21.5%[f]	–
	July 1973–June 1974	Inpatient	Los Angeles County	11.9%	21.5%	–
Los Angeles County (1977)	July 1974–June 1975	Outpatient Clinics	Los Angeles County	14.8%	21.5%	–

144

Study	Date	Facility	Location	Hispanic	Anglo	
	July 1974–June 1975	Inpatient	Los Angeles County	10.4%	21.5%	–
Los Angeles County (1978)	July 1, 1976–December 31, 1976	Outpatient Clinics	Los Angeles County	14.1%	21.5%	–
	July 1, 1976–December 31, 1976	Inpatient	Los Angeles County	9.9%	21.5%	–
Cuéllar (1977)	Fiscal Year 1976	State Hospitals	Texas	13.0%	18.5%	–
	Fiscal Year 1976	Rural Outpatient Centers	Texas	12.2%	18.5%	–
	Fiscal Year 1976	27 CMH/MR Centers	Texas catchment areas	17.9%	17.7%	+
Los Angeles County (1979)	Fiscal Year 1977/78	Outpatient Clinics	Los Angeles County	12.8%	21.5%	–
	Fiscal Year 1977/78	Inpatient	Los Angeles County	6.7%	21.5%	–
Sanchez, Acosta, & Grosser (1979)	Fiscal Year 1977/78	24 CMHCs/Clinics	Colorado	13.9%	13.5%	+
	Fiscal Year 1977/78	2 State Hospitals	Colorado	18.7%	13.5%	+
Fiedler (1979)	Fiscal Year 1973	25 CMH/MR Centers	Texas catchment areas	5.8 per 1,000 Hispanicsg	5.6 per 1,000 Anglos	+
	Fiscal Year 1974	24 CMH/MR Centers	Texas catchment areas	7.1 per 1,000 Hispanics	7.2 per 1,000 Anglos	+

(continued)

145

Table 8.1 (continued)

Study/Report	Time Period	Facility Type	Community	Percentage of MAs[a] in Patient Population or MA Admission Rate	Percentage of MAs in Community or Admission Rate of Comparison Group	MA Utilization Status[b]
	Fiscal Year 1975	27 CMH/MR Centers	Texas catchment areas	7.7 per 1,000 Hispanics	8.0 per 1,000 Anglos	−
	Fiscal Year 1976	28 CMH/MR[h] Centers	Texas catchment areas	8.0 per 1,000 Hispanics	7.7 per 1,000 Anglos	+
	Fiscal Year 1977	28 CMH/MR Centers	Texas catchment areas	8.2 per 1,000 Hispanics	7.7 per 1,000 Anglos	+
	Fiscal Year 1978	29 CMH/MR Centers	Texas catchment areas	9.3 per 1,000 Hispanics	8.5 per 1,000 Anglos	+
State of Colorado (1980)	Fiscal Year 1978/79	23 CMHCs/Clinics	Colorado	14%	13.5%	+
	Fiscal Year 1978/79	2 State Hospitals	Colorado	18.7%	13.5%	+
1970s Single Institution Treviño, Bruhn, & Bunce (1979)	September 1971–September 1972	CMHC Outpatient Center	Laredo, Texas	88.2%	86.3%	+
Andrulis (1977)	1972	CMHC	San Antonio	49%	47%	+
Heiman, Burruel, & Chávez (1975)	March 1973	CMHC Outpatient Center	Tucson, Arizona	61%	46%[i]	+

146

| Flores (1978) | October 1974–February 1975 | County Out-patient Center | East Los Angeles | 79% | 74.8%j | + |
| Heiman & Kahn (1977) | Approximately 3 months—year not recorded | CMHC Inpatient Unit | Tucson, Arizona | 41% | 41% | + |

*Community mental health/mental retardation.

aMA = Mexican American

bUnderutilization (−) and representative/overutilization (+) were defined as follows: underutilization using the percentage approach—% of MAs in catchment area − % of MAs in patient population $\geq$ .01; representative/overutilization using the percentage approach—% MAs in catchment area − % MAs in patient population < .01; underutilization using admission rates—Anglo-American (AA) admission rate − MA admission rate $\geq$ 1 per 10,000; representative/overutilization using admission rates—AA admission rate − MA admission rate < 1 per 10,000.

cFigures calculated from Table 21.2.

dFigures calculated from Table 7.1.

eAlthough no catchment area figure was provided, the authors stated that the patient population was representative of the community. This assessment is consistent with a follow-up utilization study of the same facility (Flores, 1978).

fPopulation percentages for Los Angeles County reports (1975, 1977, 1978, 1979) were obtained from Los Angeles County (1978).

gGiven that persons of Mexican origin comprised 88% of the Spanish-origin population in Texas (U.S. Census Bureau, 1973), Fiedler's study of Hispanic utilization rates was included in this review.

hIt is unknown why there is a discrepancy between the number of facilities reported by Cuéllar (27) and Fiedler (28) for the same fiscal year.

iThis figure was obtained from National Institute of Mental Health (Reference Note 6).

jThis figure was obtained from Los Angeles County (1973).

<u>Source</u>: Compiled by author.

1950s

The two earliest studies (Jaco, 1959, 1960; Libo, Dunbar, & Warren, 1962) were limited to Texas and New Mexico and to the more severely disturbed groups, which were state hospital inpatients and psychotics. Table 8.1 presents the findings of these studies. The notion that Mexican-Americans underutilize mental health services was not consistently supported. As originally noted by Barrera (1978), private facilities were underutilize in Jaco's study, but public facilities were used at almost equivale rates by Mexican-Americans and Anglo-Americans. The New Mexico study also did not support the underutilization notion. Thus, the only documented underutilization during the 1950s pertained to private facilities in Texas.

1960s

This decade marked an increase in the number of reports and studies of Mexican-American usage of mental health services. The statistical reports cited by Karno and Edgerton (1969) clearly indicated that Mexican-Americans were underrepresented across California outpatient, inpatient, and state hospital facilities for the time periods reported. Bloom (1975) also reported significant underutilization for inpatient services in Pueblo County, Colorado Unlike these two multiple institution studies, underutilization was not consistently found among those reports focusing on single institutions. Equal or overutilization rates were found for two of six individual facilities (Karno & Morales, 1971; Wignall & Koppin, 1967). Underutilization was supported by the remaining four individual reports (Karno, 1966; Philippus, 1971; Pokorny & Frazier, 1966; Torrey, 1972). In sum, the bulk of the data indicated that Mexican-Americans underutilized services across different facilities in California, Colorado, and Texas. However, Mexican-Americans were not consistently underrepresented during the 1960s.

1970s

During this decade, the quality of Mexican-American utiliza-tion research improved considerably. Statistical reports of a few geographical locales gave way to more systematic research of several regions. For the first time, the relationship of utilization to critical variables (for example, staffing patterns and diagnostic categories) was assessed. A second major improvement was that states and counties began collecting and making utilizatio data available for in-depth analysis. Sue (1977), Fiedler (1979), and Sánchez et al. (1979) were among those who made use of available data bases in the greater Seattle area, and the states of Texas and Colorado respectively.

Results of these 1970 studies showed that there were a growing number of facilities in which Mexican-Americans were proportionately represented (see Table 8.1). Of the 12 multiple facility studies, six indicated that at least some of the mental health facilities under study (primarily community mental health centers and public services) were not underutilized (Bloom, 1975; Cuéllar, 1978; Fiedler, 1979; Kruger, 1974; Sánchez et al., 1979; State of Colorado, 1980). Equal or overutilization was also reported for each of the five single institution studies.

Conclusion

There is equivocal support for the underutilization notion during each of the decades. This is clearly illustrated in Table 8.2, where the utilization research is summarized by decade and type of study (that is, multiple versus single institution study). In the 1960s there were seven multiple facility reports of underutilization and none of equal or overutilization. However, in the 1970s, of the 27 groups of facilities under study, 11 were at least proportionately utilized by Mexican-Americans. The deviation from underutilization is most clearly seen in the single institution studies and reports. In the 1960s there were four reports of underutilization and two of representative usage. In contrast, the 1970 studies reported no facilities with underutilization and five with at least proportional representation. Taking into account the available research and statistical reports, it is clear that there is no "well-documented" underutilization of mental health services by Mexican-Americans.

The findings, however, do not indicate that Mexican-Americans are now using or have ever used mental health services in parity with their representation as a total group in the southwestern United States.[4] The studies have never been representative of the total southwestern U.S. population, despite the increase in the number of locales under study. Other than Texas and Colorado, systematic research of a state's utilization patterns across all facilities has been nonexistent. Furthermore, those individual centers that reported proportionate usage by Mexican-Americans may have been a biased sample; that is, centers with more favorable utilization rates may have been more amenable to having their rates reported. In sum, more representative data are needed before any conclusions can be made about Mexican-American usage of services in the Southwest. The major point of this chapter, however, is that Mexican-Americans have used and continue to use a number of mental health facilities in parity

TABLE 8.2

Summary of Utilization Reports by Decade and
Utilization Status

Decade	Underutilization	Representative or Overutilization
1950		
Multiple institutions	1	1
Single institutions	0	1
1960		
Multiple institutions	7	0
Single institutions	4	2
1970		
Multiple institutions	15	11[a]
Single institutions	0	5

[a]Both Fiedler (1979) and Cuéllar (1977) reported representative utilization rates for Texas CMH/MR centers during fiscal year 1976. These two separate reports were tabulated only once.

Note: The types of facilities reported within one multiple institution study were independently tabulated. For example, Jaco's (1959) study was recorded twice, once for private facilities and once for public facilities.

Source: Compiled by author.

with their representation in the community. The global underutilization notion, as defined in past research, is no longer warranted.

METHODOLOGICAL CONSIDERATIONS

The findings of this review have important implications for future research directions. Before these directions are identified, methodological limitations of past research are discussed in this section. Furthermore, specific recommendations are provided to deal with these limitations.

Limitations

Of most critical importance to this area of research is the accurate identification of Mexican-Americans. Many studies did not report the way in which this ethnic group was identified among the patient population. Of those studies which did, three general approaches were used: self-report, identification by Spanish surnames, and ethnic identification made by staff members. The inaccuracies relative to each of these methods can be significant. For example, in one related study, 8.9% of the new patients identified themselves as Mexican-American, whereas a review of smaller samples indicated that almost 15% had Spanish surnames (Yamamoto, James, & Palley, 1968). Yamamoto et al. (1968) speculated that some Mexican-Americans may have listed themselves as Caucasians because in the application for services, race and ethnic categories were included together as options to identify oneself. This example points out the need to distinguish between race and ethnicity, and the differences that can result given different measures of ethnic identification.

A second methodological weakness is that patterns of utilization are usually studied without regard for highly significant differences between mental health facilities. By grouping all mental health services together, the variability of utilization rates across different types of facilities can be lost. Varying usage rates have been found across facility types in a number of studies (Bloom, 1975; Cripps, 1973; Cuéllar, 1978; Jaco, 1959, 1960; Kruger, 1974).

A third limitation of this research pertains to the general classification of diagnostic categories. Only a handful of studies provided ethnic breakdowns of diagnoses. The importance of these data is illustrated by Cuéllar's (1978) study. Although community mental health and mental retardation centers in Texas had an overall proportional representation of Mexican-Americans, there was significant variability across the major diagnostic categories. Mexican-Americans were underrepresented in mental disorders and overrepresented in drug abuse and mental retardation. The differential distribution of Mexican-Americans across the diagnostic groups is an important factor in understanding utilization patterns. This is particularly so, since the likelihood of misdiagnosis is increased for Mexican-Americans (Mercer, 1973) and Spanish-speaking patients (Marcos, Urcuyo, Kesselman, & Alpert, 1973).

A fourth methodological weakness is related to the designation of catchment areas. Since comparisons of ethnic representation in the patient population and the catchment area has been the most widely used method in assessing utilization status, it is important that accurate data be obtained. Some facilities, however, may not have defined catchment areas and therefore use figures obtained from a nearby health facility (Philippus, 1971), or the county census (Karno & Edgerton, 1969) to represent an undefined catchment area. On the other hand, some centers (particularly those with a reputation for serving Mexican-Americans) have patients who reside outside the designated catchment area (for example, Flores, 1978). In both cases, precise data are not obtained since catchment area figures do not accurately represent the community from where the patient population came.

A fifth methodological limitation is the reliance on census data; census reports may not accurately represent the number of Mexican-Americans in a particular catchment area. As Hernández, Estrada, and Alvírez (1973) noted, Mexican-Americans were undercounted in the 1970 census. Also, the criterion used to identify Mexican-Americans in the census may differ from that of the reporting facilities. For example, in one study facility reports were based on Spanish surnames only, and the census data were based on Spanish surnames and language spoken by the heads of households (Bloom, 1975).

A final problem area is that the overwhelming majority of the utilization studies and reports present data on one aspect of the service delivery system, namely, admissions. As pointed out by Sue (1977) and Goodman and Siegel (1978), minority group admission patterns may significantly differ from their termination patterns. For example, there may be no differences in how minority and majority groups are admitted. However, minority group patients may have significantly higher dropout rates. Goodman and Siegel (1978) note that in order to assess the responsiveness of mental health services to minorities, the entire treatment process must be examined.

Recommendations

The following methodological recommendations are provided so that they may be considered in addressing the identified limitations of past research.

In order to accurately identify Mexican American patients, ethnic self-identification (not to be confused with racial self-identification) and a listing of the countries of origin of the patients, their parents, and grandparents are needed for future research. Patient data would then be equivalent to 1980 census data, which also has adopted ethnic self-identification (U.S. Commission on Civil Rights, 1974). The generational data would help cross-validate the self-report data as well as provide critical data with respect to the patient population.

Data should be collected and reported in relation to the distribution of the patients across diagnostic categories.

Utilization rates should be broken down by the types of facilities, that is, public, private, outpatient, inpatient, state hospitals, and so forth.

The specific methodology and potential inaccuracies should be noted when estimates are made of the percentage of Mexican-Americans within a catchment area. Special mention is also necessary when the patient population includes residents from outside the designated catchment area.

Caution should be used when citing census data; and whenever possible, data from other sources (for example, local surveys) should be used in an attempt to arrive at the most accurate figure of ethnic representation.

Utilization studies should include at least two phases of usage, such as admissions and early terminations, or admissions and readmissions.

FUTURE RESEARCH DIRECTIONS

The two major findings of this review are first, past utilization research is flawed in assessing utilization status; and second, irrespective of this limitation, there is no clear support for the notion that Mexican-Americans underutilize mental health services. Given these findings, it is recommended that future research begin to address two major questions. First, how do Mexican-Americans utilize mental health services in relation to their assessed need for such services? Second, what are the organizational characteristics of mental health services that enhance their utilization by Mexican-Americans?

Need-Based Utilization Research

In order to accurately assess the utilization status of Mexican-Americans, need-based utilization research is critically needed. To date, no such research of Mexican-Americans has been reported. A handful of utilization studies that incorporated measures of need have been conducted with other populations. The most significant aspect of need-based utilization research is the assessment of a community or group's need for mental health services. Two needs assessment approaches that appear to be the most fruitful in the study of need-based utilization are the community survey and social indicators approaches.[5]

In the community survey approach, a random sample of community residents are interviewed to assess their need for mental health services. The interviews can be based on global mental health inventories such as the Langner (1962) scale, or on inventories that identify specific diagnoses of persons identified to be in need of services. There are some conceptual and methodological difficulties with this method, particularly in defining persons in need. Nonetheless, community surveys, specificall epidemiological research that identifies diagnostic categories, may be the most precise needs assessments approach (Weissman & Klerman, 1978).

The social indicators approach is a second type of needs assessment that can be fruitfully used in the study of need-based utilization. This approach adheres to the assumption that the need for mental health services can be inferred from sociodemographic indexes (for example, population characteristics, housing conditions, and crime rates). These data are collected and analyzed with the purpose of identifying the need for services across different sectors within the catchment area. The residents need for mental health services is then assumed to correspond to their community location and identified need for services.

Once the need for services is calculated, the researcher must decide how to best incorporate the utilization data to assess the utilization status of Mexican-Americans or any other group under study. For the community survey, need-based utilization study, there are at least two ways in which utilization rates can be incorporated. First, given a large community sample, the utilization rates of the respondents can be calculated and compared to the proportion of the respondents in need (Schwab, Warheit, & Fennell, 1975). Underutilization is identified when the proportion of the respondents in need is greater than the proportion using services. A second approach compares the percentage of a specific group in need with the percentage of that group among the patient population. (Tischler, Henisz, Myers, & Boswell, 1975). If the percentage of Mexican-Americans for example, is less among the patient population than those identified to be in need of services, then Mexican-Americans would be defined as underutilizing services.

Goodman and Hoffer (1979) demonstrated ways in which the utilization status of minority groups can be studied using the social indicators approach. First, at least two sectors within a catchment area must be identified that are of equal size, represent equal levels of need, and are represented by predominantly Mexican-Americans for one area, and predominantly Anglo-

Americans for the other. Then the utilization rates of the patients from those areas can be calculated and compared. If the utilization rate from the Mexican-American area is less than the Anglo sector, then these findings would support the notion that Mexican-Americans underutilize mental health services. Another approach that can be infered from Goodman and Hoffer (1979) is one which compares two Mexican-American sectors of a catchment area with different identified needs (high versus low need). If there is no difference in the use of services by residents from the two sectors, the underutilization would again be supported.

Organizational Factors Associated with Utilization

The majority of past research that attempted to explain Mexican-American utilization behavior focused primarily on socio-cultural variables such as different perceptions of mental health and illness, reliance on folk healers, and use of extended family members. The findings of the present review indicate that there is differential utilization of mental health facilities. Consequently, the assumption that stable cultural factors account for Mexican-American utilization patterns must be rejected. Instead, the mental health facility, the surrounding community and its institutions, and the interaction of the facility and its community should be the focus of future research that attempts to explain Mexican-American utilization.

As a first step, it is recommended that research begin to systematically examine the relationship between organizational factors and utilization. Some organizational factors in need of study are accessibility via public transportation, professional background of staff, Spanish-speaking capability of staff, and ethnicity of staff and planning board. Some of these factors have been examined in prior research (Brusco, 1979; Sánchez et al., 1979); however, only two preliminary studies have examined the relationship between one of these factors and utilization (Treviño, Reference Note 3; Rodríguez, Reference Note 7). Future research that examines the relationship between utilization and organizational factors should address the following questions: Is there a cluster of organizational commonalities across a specific group of facilities that is well utilized?; and if so, Do these factors discriminate between well and poorly used facilities? The study of organizational factors is recommended because it may account for the greatest proportion of variance in Mexican-American utilization behavior. Therefore, the direct application of these findings may have the greatest impact on utilization of services by Mexican-Americans.

SOCIOPOLITICAL IMPLICATIONS

In the past, the underutilization notion has been as much a political statement to promote Mexican-American mental health concerns as a statement to summarize the utilization research. This notion has been used to argue for the development and improvement of services to this ethnic group. In part, this has meant increasing the number of bilingual/bicultural mental health personnel (Olmedo & López, 1977).

The fact that the findings of this review do not support the underutilization notion does not reduce the potential impact that this area of research can have toward the improvement of services for Mexican-Americans. On the contrary, given that there is differential usage of services, research can now move toward identifying service characteristics most appropriate for this ethnic group. Based on systematic research, guidelines can be developed and used to effectively evaluate facilities that serve Mexican-Americans or to assist in the development of new programs. Given proper support, these guidelines could then be incorporated into the regulations of the Joint Commission on Accreditation of Hospitals for both psychiatric and community mental health facilities.

The focus on institutional factors in the study of utilization is not new. Other researchers have indicated that certain organizational factors are responsible for utilization patterns (Barrera, 1978; Padilla et al., 1975). However, past adherence to the underutilization notion has left some doubt as to whether or not usage patterns are primarily due to cultural or institutional factors. For example, Keefe (1979) offers a cultural explanation for Mexican-American underutilization of services. She specifically suggests that "emic perception of mental illness and its appropriate treatment are the key to understanding clinic underutilization by Mexican Americans" (p. 111). In contrast, the findings of the present review indicate that cultural factors are not adequate in explaining this ethnic group's utilization behavior. Organizational factors are believed to be primarily responsible for Mexican-American usage of mental health facilities.

Before significant organizational factors can be identified, it is essential that a data base of Mexican-American utilization rates be available. Not all mental health facilities, counties, and states in the Southwest, however, collect and report Mexican-American utilization data. Furthermore, as of September 1980, mental health facilities receiving federal funds (for example, community mental health centers) have yet to be required at the federal level to document Hispanic usage rates. The failure to collect and report utilization data indicates a lack of responsiveness. The efforts of Colorado, Texas, Los Angeles, and King county (Washington state) in collecting and reporting ethnic breakdowns of admissions, discharges, diagnoses, and other related utilization data should be applauded and emulated. In those areas where no data are collected, action must be taken to correct this situation.

Finally, it must be noted that the ultimate objective of this area of research should be to identify ways in which mental health services can be improved for Mexican-Americans, not to identify ways in which services can be increasingly utilized. It cannot be assumed that increased usage of mental health facilities indicates improved quality of services or results in better mental health status for Mexican-Americans. The recommendation to study facilities that are being well utilized is viewed as a first step toward defining quality mental health services for Mexican-Americans. Until methods are developed to identify facilities that provide quality care for this ethnic group, clinic usage rates will serve as a means of identifying services that may be providing quality services. It is the author's hope that the study of quality mental health care for Mexican-Americans will evolve from future utilization research.

NOTES

1. Several terms have been used in the literature to identify persons of Mexican ancestry. To facilitate the presentation of several studies cited in this chapter, only one term, Mexican-American, will be used throughout this review.

2. See Roberts (1980) for a brief review of this area.

3. Related studies that were not cited are listed below with the rationale for their exclusion. Data cited by Acosta (1977), Dondero (1973), and in part Morales (1978) were covered in the Los Angeles County (1973, 1975) statistical reports. The report by the Colorado Commission on Spanish-Surnamed Citizens (Reference Note 1), which was cited by Barrera (1978), Moustafa and Weiss (Reference Note 2), and Weaver (1973), was not available. Bachrach (1975) was not included since there was no breakdown of Mexican-Americans. Wolkon, Moriwaki, Mandel, Archuleta, Bunje, and Zimmermann (1974) provided an ethnic breakdown of those who contacted a child guidance clinic, but the study had no specific data on the utilization of services by ethnic group. Treviño (Reference Note 3) was not included since the reported utilization rates were included in Fiedler's

(1979) report. Rogawski and Edmundson (1971) investigated referrals to psychiatric outpatient facilities rather than actual utilization. Lastly, Espinoza (1979) did not collect data with respect to utilization rates.

4. The conclusions are limited to the Southwest since all but one study (Sue, 1977) pertained to southwestern locales.

5. For a review of all needs assessment methods, see Warheit, Bell, and Schwab (1977).

REFERENCE NOTES

1. Colorado Commission on Spanish-Surnamed Citizens. The status of Spanish-surnamed citizens in Colorado. Greeley, Colo.: University of Northern Colorado, Department of Political Science, 1969.

2. Moustafa, A. T., & Weiss, G. Health status and practices of Mexican Americans (Advance Report 11). Los Angeles: University of California, Mexican American Study Project, 1968.

3. Treviño, F. M. Community mental health center staffing patterns and their impact on Hispanic use of services. Paper presented at the Hispanic Health Services Research Conference, Albuquerque, New Mexico, September 1979. (Available from University of Texas Medical Branch, Galveston, Texas 77550.)

4. Wignall, C. M., & Koppin, L. L. Mexican American usage of state mental hospital facilities. Unpublished manuscript, 1966.

5. Torrey, E. F. The irrelevancy of traditional mental health services for Mexican Americans. Paper presented at the American Orthopsychiatric Association meeting, San Francisco, 1970.

6. National Institute of Mental Health. The representation of Spanish heritage populations within community mental health center catchment areas. Unpublished data, Division of Biometry, undated.

7. Rodríguez, A. Chicano staffing patterns and Chicano admissions: Is there a relationship? Unpublished manuscript, 1980. (Available from Division of Mental Health, 3520 West Oxford Avenue, Denver, Colorado 80236.)

REFERENCES

Acosta, F. X. Ethnic variables in psychotherapy: The Mexican American. In J. L. Martínez, Jr. (Ed.), Chicano psychology. New York: Academic Press, 1977.

Acosta, F. X. Barriers between mental health services and Mexican Americans: An examination of a paradox. American Journal of Community Psychology, 1979, 7, 503-20.

Andrulis, D. P. Ethnicity as a variable in the utilization and referral patterns of a comprehensive mental health center. Journal of Community Psychology, 1977, 5, 231-37.

Bachrach, L. L. Utilization of state and county mental hospitals by Spanish-Americans in 1972 (NIMH, Division of Biometry, Statistical Note 116). Washington, D.C.: U.S. Government Printing Office, 1975.

Barrera, M., Jr. Mexican-American mental health service utilization: A critical examination of some proposed variables. Community Mental Health Journal, 1978, 14, 35-45.

Bloom, B. L. Changing patterns of psychiatric care. New York: Human Sciences Press, 1975.

Brusco, B. A. Boards and councils of the Texas department of mental health and mental retardation. San Antonio: Inter-cultural Development Research Association, 1979.

Cripps, T. H. Sex, ethnicity, and admission status as determinants of patients' movement in mental health treatment. American Journal of Community Psychology, 1973, 1, 248-57.

Cuéllar, I. The utilization of mental health facilities by Mexican Americans: A test of the underutilization hypothesis. Ph.D. dissertation, University of Texas, 1977. Dissertation Abstracts International, 1978, 38, 3364-65B (University Microfilms No. 77-29,012).

Dondero, A. Los Angeles county mental health services to the Chicano population. Ph.D. dissertation, California School of Professional Psychology, 1973. Dissertation Abstracts International, 1973-74, 34, 5164B (University Microfilms No. 74-7926).

Espinoza, J. A. The underutilization of mental health services by Mexican American males. Ph.D. dissertation, United States International University, 1977. Dissertation Abstracts International, 1979, 39, 5546-5547B (University Microfilms No. 7906819).

Fiedler, F. P. Utilization, staffing and community profiles: Community mental health mental retardation centers in Texas. San Antonio: Intercultural Development Research Association, 1979.

Flores, J. L. The Utilisation of a community mental health service by Mexican Americans. International Journal of Social Psychiatry, 1978, 24, 271-75.

Goodman, A. B., & Hoffer, A. Ethnic and class factors affecting mental health clinic service usage. Evaluation and Program Planning, 1979, 2, 159-71.

Goodman, A. B., & Siegel, C. Differences in white-nonwhite community mental health center service utilization patterns. Journal of Evaluation and Program Planning, 1978, 1, 51-63.

Heiman, E. M., Burruel, G., & Chávez, N. Factors determining effective psychiatric outpatient treatment for Mexican-Americans. Hospital and Community Psychiatry, 1975, 26, 515-17.

Heiman, E. M., & Kahn, M. W. Mexican-American and European-American psychopathology and hospital course. Archives of General Psychiatry, 1977, 34, 167-70.

Hernández, J., Estrada, L., & Alvírez, D. Census data and the problem of conceptually defining the Mexican American population. Social Science Quarterly, 1973, 53, 671-87.

Jaco, E. G. Mental health of the Spanish American in Texas. In M. K. Opler (Ed.), Culture and mental health: Cross-cultural studies. New York: Macmillan, 1959.

Jaco, E. G. The social epidemiology of mental disorders. New York: Russell Sage Foundation, 1960.

Karno, M. The enigma of ethnicity in a psychiatric clinic. Archives of General Psychiatry, 1966, 14, 516-20.

Karno, M., & Edgerton, R. B. Perception of mental illness in a Mexican-American community. Archives of General Psychiatry, 1969, 20, 233-38.

Karno, M., & Morales, A. A community mental health service for Mexican-Americans in a metropolis. Comprehensive Psychiatry, 1971, 12, 116-21.

Keefe, S. E. Mexican Americans' underutilization of mental health clinics: an evaluation of suggested explanations. Hispanic Journal of Behavioral Sciences, 1979, 1, 93-115.

Kruger, D. The relationship of ethnicity to utilization of community mental health centers. Ph.D. dissertation, University of Texas at Austin, 1974. Dissertation Abstracts International, 1974, 35, 1295A (University Microfilms No. 74-24,887).

Langner, T. S. A twenty-two item screening score of psychiatric symptoms indicating impairment. Journal of Health and Human Behavior, 1962, 8, 269-76.

Libo, L. M., Dunbar, R. L., & Warren, M. M. A study of admissions to the New Mexico state hospital 1958 and 1959. Santa Fe: New Mexico Department of Public Health, Division of Mental Health, 1962.

Los Angeles County. Patient and service statistics (Report No. 10). Los Angeles: County of Los Angeles, Department of Health Services, Mental Health Services, 1973.

Los Angeles County, 1973-74 Patient and service statistics (Report No. 11). Los Angeles: County of Los Angeles, Department of Health Services, Mental Health Services, 1975.

Los Angeles County. Client and service statistics: 1974-75 (Report No. 12). Los Angeles: County of Los Angeles, Department of Health Services, Mental Health Services, 1977.

Los Angeles County. Plan for mental health services 1978-79/ 1978-81. Los Angeles: County of Los Angeles, Department of Health Services, Mental Health Services, 1978.

Los Angeles County. Plan for mental health services 1979-80/ 1979-82. Los Angeles: County of Los Angeles, Department of Mental Health, 1979.

Marcos, L. R., Urcuyo, L., Kesselman, M., Alpert, M. The language barrier in evaluating Spanish-American patients. Archives of General Psychiatry, 1973, 29, 655-59.

Mercer, J. R. Labelling the mentally retarded. Berkeley: University of California, 1973.

Morales, A. The need for nontraditional mental health programs in the "barrio." In J. M. Casas & S. E. Keefe (Eds.), Family and mental health in the Mexican American community (Monograph No. 7). Los Angeles: University of California, Spanish Speaking Mental Health Research Center, 1978.

Olmedo, E. L., & López, S. (Eds.). Hispanic mental health professionals (Monograph No. 5). Los Angeles: University of California, Spanish Speaking Mental Health Research Center, 1977.

Padilla, A. M., & Ruiz, R. A. Latino mental health: A review of the literature (DHEW Publication No. (HSM) 73-9143). Washington, D.C.: U.S. Government Printing Office, 1973.

Padilla, A. M., Ruiz, R. A., & Álvarez, R. Community mental health services for the Spanish-speaking/surnamed population. American Psychologist, 1975, 30, 892-905.

Philippus, M. J. Successful and unsuccessful approaches to mental health services for an urban Hispano-American population. American Journal of Public Health, 1971, 61, 820-30.

Pokorny, A. D., & Frazier, S. Report of the administrative survey of Texas state mental hospitals, 1966. Austin: Texas Department of Mental Health/Mental Retardation, 1966.

Roberts, R. E. Prevalence of psychological distress among Mexican Americans. Journal of Health and Social Behavior, 1980, 21, 134-45.

Rogawski, A., & Edmundson, B. Factors affecting the outcome of psychiatric interagency referral. American Journal of Psychiatry, 1971, 127, 925-34.

Sánchez, A., Acosta, F., & Grosser, R. Mental health services to ethnic minorities in Colorado. Denver: Division of Mental Health, Department of Institutions, State of Colorado, 1979.

Schwab, J. J., Warheit, G. J., & Fennell, E. B. An epidemiologic assessment of needs and utilization of services. Evaluation, 1975, 2, Vol. 2, 65-67.

State of Colorado. Client characteristics for all admission episodes FY 1978-79 (Evaluation Report No. 26). Denver: State of Colorado, Department of Institutions, Division of Mental Health, 1980.

Sue, S. Community mental health services to minority groups: Some optimism, some pessimism. American Psychologist, 1977, 32, 616-24.

Tischler, G. L., Henisz, J. E., Myers, J. K., & Boswell, P. C. Utilization of Mental Health Services: I. Patienthood and the prevalence of symptomology in the community. Archives of General Psychiatry, 1975, 32, 411-15.

Torrey, E. F. The mind game: Witchdoctors and psychiatrists. New York: Bantam Books, 1972.

Treviño, F. M., Bruhn, J. G., & Bunce, H., III. Utilization of community mental health services in a Texas-Mexico border city. Social Science and Medicine, 1979, 13A, 331-34.

U.S. Census Bureau. Census of population: 1970. Subjects Reports. Persons of Spanish origin (PC(2)-1C). Washington, D.C.: U.S. Dept. of Commerce, 1973.

U.S. Commission on Civil Rights. Counting the forgotten: The 1970 census count of persons of Spanish speaking background in the United States. Washington, D.C.: U.S. Government Printing Office, 1974.

Warheit, G. J., Bell, R. A., Schwab, J. J. Needs assessment approaches: Concepts and methods (DHEW Publication No. ADM 77-472.) Washington, D.C.: U.S. Government Printing Office, 1977.

Weaver, J. L. Mexican-American health care behavior: A critical review of the literature. Social Science Quarterly, 1973, 54, 85-102.

Weissman, M. M., & Klerman, G. L. Epidemiology of mental disorders: Emerging trends in the United States. Archives of General Psychiatry, 1978, 35, 705-12.

Wignall, C. M., & Koppin, L. L. Mexican-American usage of state mental hospital facilities. Community Mental Health Journal, 1967, 3, 137-48.

Wolkon, G. H., Moriwaki, S., Mandel, S. M., Archuleta, Jr.,
Bunje, P., & Zimmermann, S. Ethnicity and social class in
the delivery of services: analysis of a child guidance clinic.
American Journal of Public Health, 1974, 64, 709-812.

Yamamoto, J., James, Q. C., & Palley, N. Cultural problems
in psychiatric therapy. Archives of General Psychiatry,
1968, 19, 45-49.

9

EVALUATION OF A BILINGUAL BICULTURAL TREATMENT PROGRAM FOR MEXICAN-AMERICAN PSYCHIATRIC INPATIENTS

Israel Cuéllar, Lorwen C. Harris, and Nancy Naron

A long-standing concern in the area of mental health service delivery has been the need to develop services that are sufficiently flexible to respond to individuals of diverse cultural backgrounds. A growing body of literature has been developed that examines the differential utilization of mental health facilities and services by different socioeconomic, cultural, and ethnic minority groups (Hollingshead & Redlich, 1958; Giordano & Giordano, 1976; Sanua, 1966; Rabkin & Streuning, 1975; Padilla & Ruiz, 1973). A substantial portion of this literature indicates that some minority groups are significantly underserved while others are inappropriately served; in either case, the needs of particular segments of our society are not adequately addressed or considered in the design and implementation of human service delivery systems.

Giordano and Giordano (1976) conclude that "too many programs now in existence are out of touch with the real needs of the people they are designed to serve" (p. 12). Both the underutilization and the inappropriate use of mental health services by Mexican-Americans have been attributed, in part, to the notion that traditional services are irrelevant or incompatible with the needs of Mexican-Americans (Padilla, Ruiz, & Alvarez, 1975; Torrey, 1972; Ramírez, 1980). The President's Commission

---

The authors wish to express their appreciation to the Hogg Foundation for Mental Health of the University of Texas at Austin for making funds available to conduct the evaluation and for its encouragement and consultation throughout the project. Many thanks are also due to the staff members of the San Antonio State Hospital who contributed their time to the successful completion of this study.

on Mental Health in its subtask panel report on the mental health
of Hispanic Americans called for a recognition of the unique
linguistic and sociocultural needs of Hispanics and for the inclusion of relevant linguistic and sociocultural elements in mental
health service delivery systems where applicable, that is, where
significant numbers of persons with limited English-speaking
ability reside within a service area:

> A mental health program which attempts to reduce
> a patient's anxieties with medication or individual
> therapy while neglecting or assaulting their socio-
> cultural values will defeat its own purpose and
> cause more damage than benefit. In short, individ-
> uals have their roots in their ethnicity. Damage to
> those ethnic roots can cause serious psychological
> trauma, while respect for them facilitates the develop-
> ment of a therapeutic alliance and healing process.
> (p. 910)

Despite the apparent interest and the demand for culturally
sensitive treatment programs, there have been no published
articles reporting systematic outcome data on culturally responsive
inpatient treatment programs for Mexican-Americans. This chapter reports the preliminary results of the evaluation of a unique
bilingual/bicultural treatment program for Spanish-speaking,
Mexican-American psychiatric patients. It reports a study of
Mexican-American psychotic patients who were either served
within a bilingual/bicultural treatment milieu (experimental group)
or were treated within a more traditional milieu (control group).
A description of the program, the patients served, the patients'
involvement, and their outcome characteristics are examined in
detail.

RESEARCH METHODS

Bilingual/Bicultural Treatment Program

The Bilingual/Bicultural Treatment Program at the San
Antonio State Hospital in San Antonio, Texas, is an inpatient
unit that in the past has been operated with both federal and
state funds and staffed exclusively with bilingual/bicultural
personnel of Mexican-American heritage. It is a specialized
unit for the treatment of Mexican-American psychiatric patients,
most of whom are schizophrenic. The program emphasizes the

use of linguistic and cultural elements in the treatment of Spanish-speaking, Mexican-American psychiatric patients. Most of the ward conversation and treatment activities are conducted in Spanish or English and Spanish, and specific customs and beliefs characteristic of Chicanos are integrated into the treatment process. The ward decor reflects this ethnic theme and is designed to facilitate treatment for Mexican-American psychiatric patients, reducing the cultural shock and isolation believed to be experienced by Mexican-American patients in state hospitals. The program serves 60 patients on a daily basis and between 150 and 200 adult patients yearly.

In many ways the program activities are quite similar to activities of other inpatient units throughout the hospital. For example, clinical activities include chemotherapy, individual therapy, group therapy, community meetings, family therapy, behavior modification, and a privilege-level system. Other ward activities include social and recreational programming and occupational therapy. Referral sources are used for a broad range of rehabilitative services that include vocational evaluation, training, and education. The main differences between program activities conducted in the bilingual/bicultural treatment program and those conducted in other inpatient units of the hospital are that the activities are conducted by Mexican-American staff in Spanish and English, as required by the patient, and cultural elements are included to enhance effectiveness.

Comparison of Experimental and Control Wards

During the time of the present study (1979–80), the experimental ward, a bilingual/bicultural treatment ward, had an average daily census of 54.33 patients. There were four control wards that had a combined average daily census of 55.49 patients. The average number of nursing staff actually on duty (exclusive of occupational therapy, recreation, social work, psychology, and medical staff) on the experimental ward during the 7 A.M-3 P.M. shift was 7.58. The average number of nursing staff actually on duty in the control wards during the 7-3 shift was 8.36. On the experimental ward the number of nursing staff dropped to 5.66 during the evening shift (3-11) and decreased to 3.8 on the night shift. On the control wards the average number of nursing staff for the evening shift was 5.83 and 4.71 for the night shift. The overall average for all three shifts on the control wards was 9.32 patients per nursing staff member, while for the experimental ward the overall average was 10.34 patients per nursing staff member.

On the experimental ward, 100 percent of the staff and patients were bilingual and of Mexican heritage. On the control wards the percentage of patients and staff of Mexican heritage was between 22 percent and 46 percent throughout the duration of the study.

The main differences, aside from the experimental conditions, between the control and experimental wards were not the average daily census or average number of nursing staff on duty. Rather, the differences were that the control wards were admittin wards with more professional staff (social workers and psychiatrists in particular) and had a much higher turnover rate in patients. The experimental ward, on the other hand, had a more stable population in that it is not an admitting unit, as are the control units, and approximately half of the patients are chronic. The physical design of the buildings was identical for all wards involved in the study. Each ward, however, had its individual interior decor.

Characteristics of the Sample

The subjects were patients admitted to the Adult Psychiatri Unit of the San Antonio State Hospital during the period of Febru ary 1, 1979, through March 31, 1980. Patients were randomly assigned to the experimental and control groups. The criteria for eligibility in the study were that the patients be psychotic, Mexican-American, and Spanish-speaking. Patients with a primary diagnosis of mental retardation, organic brain syndrome, alcohol or drug abuse, or a personality disorder were omitted from the study. Eligible patients were randomly selected and assigned to the experimental and control groups. A total of 82 Mexican-American psychiatric patients were selected for the study. Characteristics of the sample were as follows: 56.1 percent were males and 43.9 percent were females; the average age was 34.5 years; the majority (93.5 percent) were Catholic and 5.2 percent were Protestant. A breakdown of patients into marital status categories revealed that: 53.7 percent had never married, 11.0 percent were separated, 3.7 percent were widowed, 11 percent were divorced, and 19.5 percent were married. Approximately 66.8 percent were from urban areas. Most (64 percent) were on some type of court commitment; 2.6 percent were on an emergency commitment; 31 percent were voluntary patients and 1.3 percent were on an indefinite commitment. Most had been previously admitted to the San Antonio State Hospital. Only 21 percent of the patients were first admissions. The

average number of previous admissions for the group was 3.4,
with a range of 0 to 14. Most (61 percent) of the patients had
received previous outpatient care. The majority of the patients
were either unemployed, unable to work, or were not in the
labor force (76 percent). Only 5.2 percent were employed on
a full-time basis and 3.9 percent were employed on a part-time
basis. The group as a whole had an average of eight years of
education; however, 33.8 percent of the group had between 10
and 12 years of education and 5.2 percent had some college.
Approximately 29 percent of the group had less than six years
of education. The majority of the patients reported their usual
living situation as being with their family (62.3 percent); 11.7
percent reported living alone and 10.4 percent reported living
with their spouses. Although only one patient reported not being
a U.S. citizen, several patients were thought to be illegal aliens.
Language abilities were as follows: 19.5 percent reported speaking
Spanish only and 75.3 percent reported they spoke both Spanish
and English. Although 3.4 percent reported on their intake
forms that they spoke English only, all subjects were known to
speak some Spanish. The most common diagnosis for the patients
was schizophrenia, chronic undifferentiated type, which represented 39 percent of the cases. The second most common diagnosis was schizophrenia, paranoid type, which described 22
percent of the patients. The remainder of the diagnoses were
manic depressive illnesses (depressed, manic, and cyclic types),
psychotic depression, acute schizophrenic episode, latent schizophrenia, and schizophrenia in remission.

Sources of Data and Terms Defined

The data sources were the Problem Oriented Record System
(PORS), the Psychotic Inpatient Profile (PIP), the Socialization
Level Scale (SLS), and the Work Level Scale (WLS) of the Social
Adjustment Behavior Rating Scale (SABRS) and the Acculturation
Rating Scale for Mexican Americans (ARSMA). These sources
are described below.

The Problem Oriented Record System (PORS) is a uniform
record-keeping system used throughout all state hospitals in
Texas. It is designed to provide important demographic, clinical,
social, and rehabilitation data to pinpoint patient problems that
must be remedied in the treatment process. It is designed to
simplify evaluations of treatment by defining each problem, its
particular treatment, and the goal to be accomplished with regard
to each problem. This record system has been in operation at

the San Antonio State Hospital since 1978. A wide range of social, demographic, clinical, and process data were collected from the PORS record on all subjects. Some data were used exactly as recorded while other data were grouped, weighted, or classified (see terms defined).

The Psychotic Inpatient Profile (PIP) is a behavior inventor designed to measure 12 dimensions or syndromes of currently observable psychotic behavior: excitement, hostility, paranoia, anxiety, retardation, seclusiveness, care needed, psychotic disorganization, grandiosity, perceptual distortion, depression, and disorientation (Lorr & Vestre, 1969). The PIP consists of 74 statements descriptive of manifest ward behavior and 22 statements descriptive of patient self-reports. The inventory is completed by a nurse or psychiatric aide following three days of observation and interaction with the patient. Each statement is noted on a continuum ranging from "not at all" to "nearly always." The rated statements are then summed and converted to a t-score for each subscale. T-scores of the subscales were averaged in this study to yield an overall mean for each patient profile.

The Social Adjustment Behavior Rating Scale is designed for inpatient psychiatric populations and is composed of two scales: the Work Level Scale and the Socialization Level Scale (Aumack, 1962). Both scales are completed by nursing staff who are familiar with the patients being assessed. The Work Level Scale (WLS) is designed to measure physical self-maintenanc and work potential, ranging from complete dependency at one extreme to an ability to maintain and support others at the other extreme. The higher the score, the more able the patient is to secure and maintain employment. The Socialization Level Scale (SLS) measures adequacy of social interaction ranging from complete social isolation at one extreme to maximal breadth and depth of mature social interaction at the other extreme. Similar to the WLS, the SLS indicates a higher level of social functioning the higher the score. Both scales have been developed with psychiatric patients and have established reliability and validity (Aumack, 1962).

The Acculturation Rating Scale for Mexican Americans (ARSMA) is a behavioral acculturation scale composed of 20 items. Normative data were collected from normal and psychiatric Mexican-American populations. The ARSMA yields a measure of acculturation between 1 and 5 on a continuum on which 1 represents a Mexican-oriented individual, 2 represents a Mexican-oriented bicultural, 3 represents an equal bicultural, 4 represents an Anglo-oriented bicultural, and 5 represents a very Anglicized Mexican-American. Its reliability and validity have been demonstrated to be sufficient (Cuéllar, Harris & Jasso, 1980).

Terminology

Initial severity—At the time of initial staffing, severity
of a patient's psychiatric and social problems was determined by
a multidisciplinary treatment team. Severity was indicated on a
7-point scale from (1) not evident, (2) very mild to (7) extremely
severe.

Severity at discharge—A patient's primary psychiatric
and primary social problems, if any, were rated as to severity
on a 7-point scale (see initial severity) at time of discharge by
the treatment team or one of its members.

Psychiatric goal accomplished—This is the extent of goal
accomplished in regard to the primary psychiatric problem at time
of discharge. Goal accomplished is rated as (1) none, (2) partially, or (3) totally.

Chronicity measure—Total length of stay was entered into
a step-wise regression equation as the criterion variable. Five
variables (number of previous admissions, education level,
present length of stay, diagnosis, and age) were selected through
factor analysis and entered as predictor variables. Beta weights,
yielded by the regression analysis, were used to weight the
predictor variables that were summed with the total length of
stay to produce a composite chronicity measure for each subject.

Medication at one month—Antipsychotic medication and
dosage were recorded for each subject after one month of hospitalization. The dosage was converted into Thorazine equivalent
units (Hollister, 1973) and then placed in a ratio to the subject's
weight (equivalent mg. of Thorazine/weight in kg.).

Medication at discharge—Antipsychotic medication level
upon release from the hospital was recorded and converted to a
ratio of mg. of Thorazine to weight (same procedure as used for
medication at one month).

Improvement in primary psychiatric problem—The rated
severity of a subject's psychiatric problem upon discharge (7-
point scale from "not evident" to "extremely severe") was subtracted from the severity rating given at the initial staffing to
yield an improvement score. (The primary psychiatric problem
was the problem noted in staffing as deserving the most emphasis
in treatment.)

Procedure

All eligible patients were assigned a random number that
determined their inclusion or exclusion from the study and their
status as either a control or experimental patient. Patients

assigned to the control wards remained on one of four acute-care wards to which they had been admitted. Patients randomly assigned to the experimental Bilingual/Bicultural ward were transferred from the admitting ward to the experimental ward within two to ten days after admission with the average being about five days after admission. The initial stay on the admitting ward was required in order to determine diagnosis and eligibility for possible inclusion in the study. Medication and dosage, definition of presenting problems and the treatment plan were also established on the admission units prior to the experimental patient's transfer to the Bilingual/Bicultural ward.

The randomization procedure created an experimental group that was substantially equivalent to the control group with the exception that the control subjects remained on the same ward to which they had been admitted, while the experimental group was transferred to another ward after a very brief stay on the admitting ward. A total of 160 subjects were randomly selected to participate in the study. Of these, 41 were assigned to the experimental group and 41 to the control group. Patients who left against medical advice or were discharged within three weeks of admission were excluded from the study in order to allow for an adequate period of exposure to the experimental condition. A total of 87 subjects, 45 in the control group and 42 in the experimental group, were eliminated from the study on this basis. The first 41 experimental and first 41 control subjects who remained at least one month in treatment comprised the 82 subjects analyzed in this evaluation.

Data were collected on patients at three points in time: at the time of admission, after four weeks of hospitalization, and at time of discharge. After initial staffing, a psychiatric aide or social worker assigned to a particular experimental or control patient was asked to rate the patient on the PIP and on the SLS and the WLS. After one month of hospitalization, a staff member again rated the patient in terms of psychopathology (PIP), socialization, and work functioning. PORS data such as number of seclusions, number of off-ground passes, number of hours of secluded and attended activities, and level of psychotropic medications were also gathered on the patient at this time. Upon discharge, the level of psychotropic medication, the degree of psychiatric and social goals accomplished, and the present and total lengths of hospitalization were obtained. These data were collected by psychology graduate students employed part time. They administered the standardized questionnaires (PIP, WLS, and SLS) to the psychiatric attendants, social workers, and case managers and administered the ARSMA to the patients.

RESULTS OF THE STUDY

The goal of this evaluation was to determine the efficacy of culturally sensitive milieu treatment for Mexican-American psychotic inpatients. In order to assess the treatment efficacy, the experimental and control groups were compared in terms of the aforementioned measures of pathology, socialization, potential for employment, acquired ward privileges, number of seclusions, and off-ground passes, and frequency of use of rehabilitative services. In addition, the relationships among these measures and descriptive data were examined to uncover correlates and patterns.

Social Adjustment and Pathology

The relationship between severity of the psychotic disorder and level of social functioning was examined and found to be significant. Patients whose social functioning and interactions, as measured by the SLS, were perceived as most inadequate were those who obtained the highest scores on the PIP. Administration of the PIP subscales after one month of hospitalization revealed Paranoia, Anxiety, Retardation, Seclusiveness, Care Needed, Psychotic Disorganization, Depression, and Disorientation subscales to be significantly correlated with the SLS scores, such that the more severe the psychopathology, the less adequate was the social functioning (see Table 9.1). The correlation obtained for all subjects between the SLS and the mean score on the PIP was $r = -.63$, $p < .001$. The strong relationship found between social impairment and psychiatric impairment evident for the entire group was also found for the experimental and control groups when examined separately (see Table 9.1).

Another significant relationship found was between work level and the severity of psychotic behavior, as measured by the WLS and PIP respectively; the more dependent a patient, the greater was the pathology as measured by the PIP. The PIP subscales, Anxiety, Retardation, Seclusiveness, Care Needed, Psychotic Disorganization, and Disorientation were each negatively correlated with the WLS ($p < .05$) for all subjects, as well as for the experimental and control groups when individually examined. Work level, like socialization level, was highly correlated with the mean PIP score ($r = .85$, $p < .001$), and each tended to correlate with the same subscales on the PIP. These significant correlations were all negative: the greater the extent of pathology the lower the work or social functioning of the patient.

TABLE 9.1

Significant Psychotic Profile Correlates of Social Level in the Sample

Social Level Correlates on PIP[a]	Combined Group n = 82		Experimental Group n = 41		Control Group n = 41	
	r	p	r	p	r	p
Excitement	ns*		ns		ns	
Hostility	ns		ns		ns	
Paranoia	-.31	.002	-.27	.041	-.29	.030
Anxiety	-.45	.001	-.39	.006	-.55	.001
Retardation	-.56	.001	-.46	.001	-.61	.001
Seclusiveness	-.75	.001	-.69	.001	-.80	.001
Care Needed	-.60	.001	-.61	.001	-.62	.001
Psychotic disorganization	-.58	.001	-.56	.001	-.53	.001
Grandiosity	ns		ns		ns	
Depression	-.26	.008	ns		-.38	.007
Perceptual disorganization	ns		ns		ns	
Disorientation	-.41	.001	-.47	.001	-.37	.010
Positive elevations[b]	-.58	.001	-.62	.001	-.44	.002
Minus elevations[c]	.58	.001	.50	.001	.54	.001
PIP mean score	-.63	.001	-.65	.001	-.54	.001

*Not significant.
[a]PIP = psychotic inpatient profile.
[b]Positive elevation = total number of standard deviations above the mean for all 12 subscales of PIP.
[c]Minus elevation = total number of standard deviations below the mean on all 12 subscales of PIP.
Source: Compiled by authors.

An examination of the mean scores obtained for the experimental and control subjects on the PIP, the SLS, and the WLS indicated that the two groups were not significantly different at admission or after one month in treatment (see Table 9.2). The mean scores on the PIP, SLS, and WLS all indicated that the patients in both the experimental group and the control group improved after one month of hospitalization; however, the changes as measured by these standardized instruments were small and not statistically significant.

Severity of pathology. Multiple measures of severity of pathology were gathered. Measures other than the PIP were severity ratings of the patient's primary psychiatric problem at admission and again at discharge. Severity of the primary psychiatric problem upon admission and at discharge was not significantly correlated with the PIP mean score obtained after one month of hospitalization. Furthermore, no significant differences were found between the experimental and control groups in terms of severity either upon admission or discharge. However, other measures of pathology taken at different times during the course of hospitalization were found to correlate in numerous instances with several variables. In general, the more severely disturbed patients, as measured by the PIP, were more likely to function at lower levels of social and work adjustment, have a greater length of hospitalization, require more seclusion, and were generally younger in age.

Treatment Trends

Present length of stay

The average length of stay for patients in the experimental group was 81 days, with the median being 63 days. The control group's median stay was 51 days. Group differences were nonsignificant. The total length of stay (duration of all previous hospitalization plus present stay) was also not significantly different for the experimental and control groups. However, different factors were found to be correlated with length of stay for the two groups. Patients who remained in treatment longer in the experimental program were more likely to be chronic (r = .42, p = .004), and to demonstrate more retardation (r = .42, p = .003), and seclusiveness (r = .28, p = .035). Patients in the control group who remained longer in treatment exhibited higher levels of anxiety (r = .33, p = .015). In both groups, weekend and overnight passes were associated with reduced lengths of stay (r = -.31, p = .026). In the control group, the

TABLE 9.2

Differences between Admission and after One Month of Hospitalization

Variable	N	Mean at Admission	Mean at 1 Month	Mean Difference	T Value	2-Tail Probability
			Combined Group			
PIP mean	33	48.8727	45.3091	-3.5636	-2.07	.046
Social level	33	20.5152	21.6667	1.1515	.61	.545
Work level	33	17.3333	19.3030	1.9697	1.60	.120
			Experimental Group			
PIP mean	17	47.0412	45.3118	-1.7294	-.95	.357
Social level	17	23.4706	24.4118	.9412	.32	.755
Work level	17	19.5882	20.9412	1.3529	.79	.441
			Control Group			
PIP mean	16	50.8187	45.3062	-5.5125	-1.87	.082
Social level	16	17.3750	18.7500	1.375	.58	.571
Work level	16	14.9375	17.5625	2.6250	1.45	.169

Note: Differences between experimentals and controls in regard to change in PIP mean, social level, and work level over time (between admission and one month) were nonsignificant. Also, differences between experimentals and controls at admission and at one month were nonsignificant.
Source: Compiled by the authors.

more Mexican-oriented the patient with regard to acculturation, the greater the length of hospitalization (r = -.27, p = .042); this was not true for the experimental group.

Total length of stay

The median total length of hospitalization for the whole group (n = 82) was seven months; for the experimental group it was six months, and for the control group it was ten months. The average total length of stay for the whole group was 1.83 years. No significant differences were found between the experimental and control groups in relation to total length of hospitalization.

The correlates of total length of hospitalization were somewhat different from the correlates of present length of hospitalization. Patients with greater total length of stay were more likely to exhibit higher need of care and greater depression, were older, less acculturated (that is, more Mexican-oriented), less educated, and more chronic. They were also more likely to have a greater number of previous admissions, to receive lower dosages of medication and be given fewer weekend or overnight passes.

In the control group, the more Mexican-oriented the patient, the more likely they were to have greater lengths of stay, both in terms of present and total lengths of stay. In the experimental group, acculturation was not related to either present or total length of stay.

Seclusions

Most patients did not require seclusions during their first month of hospitalization, but a significant minority (32 percent) did. They were secluded because they represented an imminent danger either to themselves or to others. The average number of seclusions during their first month of hospitalization was 1.32 for all subjects. Approximately one-third of the patients secluded were secluded only once. The range, however, was from one to 30 seclusions during the first month of hospitalization. The average number of seclusions in the experimental group was 1.02 while it was 1.6 in the control; this difference was not significant.

Patients who required a greater number of seclusions were more likely to be rated as excitable (r = .22, p = .024), hostile (r = .30, p = .003), and paranoid on the PIP. Their primary psychiatric problems were more likely to be rated as severe and they obtained higher mean scores on the PIP (r = .25, p = .011).

Age, sex, and psychotropic medication level were not related to number of seclusions.

Antipsychotic Medication

For the overall sample, antipsychotic medication level at one month after hospitalization was found to be associated with age, severity of depression, level of acculturation, and total length of hospitalization. Age and medication level were correlated (r = -.23, p = .020) such that youth tended to be associated with higher dosages of medication. The less severely depressed were found to receive more antipsychotic medication (r = -.23, p = .017), as may be expected since antipsychotic medications are often not the drugs of choice for depressed patients. In assessing the relationship between level of acculturation and level of antipsychotic medication, it was found that the less acculturated patients were more likely to receive higher dosages of medication (r = .19, p = .044). In addition, medication dosages after one month in treatment and at discharge were positively correlated (r = .41, p = .004).

Several dimensions of psychotic behavior (assessed after one month) were associated with discharge medication level. For example, discharge level of medication was positively correlated with degrees of excitement (r = .32, p = .002), hostility (r = .27, p = .007), care needed (r = .21, p = .029), psychotic disorganization (r = .30, p = .003), perceptual distortion (r = .19, p = .043), and the mean PIP score (r = .27, p = .006). At the time of discharge, medication level was negatively correlated with WLS (r = -.24, p = .014) and the number of off-ground passes (r = -.31, p = .002). Of additional import is the finding that the experimental and control groups did not differ in levels of medication at discharge or after one month of hospitalization.

Rehabilitation Hours

As part of the Problem Oriented Record System (PORS), a record is kept of the number of formally scheduled and attended hours of rehabilitation therapy for each patient. As a whole, 80 percent of all patients attended at least one hour of formal occupational therapy during their fourth week of hospitalization. The average number of hours of attendance for the entire group during their fourth week was 8.4 hours. For the experimental group, it was 12.47 hours and 4.43 hours for the control group. Group differences were statistically significant ($t(77)$ = 4.98, p < .001). Based on the PORS record system, the experimental patients were scheduled for and attended significantly more hours of formal occupational therapies than did the control patients.

Improvement in Primary Psychiatric Problem

The rated severity of a patient's primary psychiatric problem at discharge was subtracted from the severity of a patient's primary psychiatric problem given at the time of initial staffing to produce an improvement score. In the overall sample, patients judged as having made the most improvement in regard to their primary psychiatric problems were those who were less seclusive, required less care, exhibited less psychotic disorganization, had the fewest previous admissions, and were less chronic (as determined by the chronicity measure described previously). Those patients with shorter lengths of stay (both present and total) also made the greatest psychiatric improvement. Patients who were judged at the initial staffing as having more severe problems were those who made the greatest improvement. Both SLS and WLS scores obtained at one month were positively correlated with degree of improvement at discharge ($\underline{r}$ = .22, $\underline{p}$ = .021 and $\underline{r}$ = .29, $\underline{p}$ = .006 respectively). In summary, the data indicated that patients who made the greatest gains were those who were less chronic, required the least care, were less seclusive, stayed in the hospital less, and functioned at higher social and work levels.

Although 78 percent of the patients in the experimental group and 68 percent in the control group were found to improve, the difference between the experimental and control groups in regard to improvement scores was not statistically significant.

Acculturation Level

An important overall consideration in the present study was the relationship between level of acculturation and treatment trends. Acculturation level was assessed with the Acculturation Rating Scale for Mexican Americans (Cuéllar et al., 1980). The mean for the group was 2.88 with a standard deviation of ±.76. There was no significant difference in level of acculturation between the experimental and control groups. The correlates of level of acculturation, however, were in some cases different for experimentals and controls (see Table 9.3). For the overall sample, it was found that the more Mexican-oriented patients tended to have longer total length of hospitalization, were older, and required higher dosages of antipsychotic medication. The more Anglicized, the higher the social and work levels were, including level of education and number of passes.

Less acculturated Mexican-Americans in the experimental group were more likely to obtain higher ratings with regard to

TABLE 9.3

Significant Correlates of Level of Acculturation in the Sample

Significant Correlates of Acculturation	Combined Group n = 82		Experimental Group n = 41		Control Group n = 41	
	r	p	r	p	r	p
Present LOS[a]	-.19	ns*		ns	-.27	.042
Total LOS[b]	.21	.041		ns	-.54	.001
Social level	.21	.028		ns		ns
Work level	.21	.026	.27	.039		ns
Psychiatric goal accomplished	ns		-.31	.037		ns
Meds[c] at 1 month	-.20	.031	-.32	.020		ns
Previous admissions						
Age	ns			ns	-.34	.013
Education	-.29	.003		ns	-.39	.005
Passes	.23	.016		ns		ns
ISPPP[d]	.19	.041		ns		ns
ISPSP[e]	ns	ns	.26	.049		ns
SPSPD[f]	ns	ns	.29	.033		ns
Chronicity	-.24	.013		ns	-.49	.001

*Not significant.

[a] Present length of stay this admission.

[b] Total length of stay for all admissions.

[c] Meds = psychotropic medication/kg. of body weight.

[d] ISPPP = Initial severity of Primary Psychiatric Problem.

[e] ISPSP = Initial severity of Primary Social Problem.

[f] SPSPD = Severity of Primary Social Problem at Discharge.

Source: Compiled by the authors.

180

degree of goals accomplished than more acculturated Mexican-Americans. (This was not so for the control group.) The more acculturated Mexican-Americans in the experimental group were rated as having less severe primary psychiatric and social problems. Less acculturated patients were also rated as having less severe social problems at discharge than were more acculturated Mexican-Americans. Additionally, less acculturated Mexican-Americans were found to demonstrate less potential for employment.

In summary, there were some very important differences in the way Mexican-Americans of differing levels of acculturation were perceived, judged, and treated within the experimental and control groups. In the control group, Mexican-American patients rated as being less acculturated (or more Mexican) were those that were older, more chronic, and had greater lengths of stay. In the experimental group, Mexican-Americans rated as being less acculturated were judged as having less severe primary psychiatric and social problems, and were more likely than more acculturated Mexican-Americans to reach their goal in regard to their primary psychiatric problems.

Chronicity

A factor analysis of all variables yielded a chronicity factor comprised of five variables: number of previous admissions, education, present length of stay, diagnosis, and age. These variables were entered into a stepwise regression equation as independent variables to predict total length of stay. The beta weights yielded by the regression analysis were used to weight the independent variables to produce the composite chronicity measure for each subject.

Only three of the subscales of the PIP (excitement, seclusiveness, and care needed) were found to be significantly correlated with chronicity. Overall, chronic patients were more likely to be seclusive, require more care, and be less excitable than acute patients. They were found to be older, less educated, less acculturated, and have lower work and social functioning. Additionally, the chronic patients tended to have more previous admissions and greater lengths of stay. They were not found, however, to be more severely psychotic.

In the experimental group, social level, work level, and acculturation were not significantly correlated with chronicity while in the control group, these were significantly correlated. However, present length of stay was positively correlated with chronicity (r = .40, p = .004) in the experimental group but not in the control group.

DISCUSSION

The findings reported are of enormous value in furthering our understanding of the psychiatric characteristics of psychotic Mexican-Americans treated at the San Antonio State Hospital. The findings also add to our understanding of the effects of a culturally relevant treatment milieu on Spanish-speaking Mexican-American psychiatric patients.

At the San Antonio State Hospital, Spanish-speaking Mexican-American psychotic patients treated in the Bilingual/Bicultural Treatment Program were found to function as well as, and in some cases better than, those treated within regular admitting units. Based on the measures used in the present study to assess psychiatric and behavioral functioning, neither the experimental nor the control wards were found to be clearly superior to the other. Measures of psychiatric, social, and work adjustment taken after one month of hospitalization indicated no significant differences between the experimental and control groups. Staff ratings of severity of pathology, psychiatric improvement, and goal accomplished at time of discharge also indicated no significant differences between gains made by patients in the experimental group and those in the control group

A major difference was found between the experimental and control groups in amount of participation in rehabilitation therapies. The experimental group was found to be significantly more involved in rehabilitation or occupational therapy and support programs than the control group. Thus, the major therapeutic effects of the bilingual/bicultural milieu were not in terms of effecting greater psychiatric improvement but were revealed in facilitation of treatment and enhancement of program involvement.

It may very well be that the main differences produced by culturally relevant treatment programming are related to quality of care characteristics such as comfort, ease of communication, shared sense of community, hope, facilitation, and so forth. These are all ingredients that one would want to include in a treatment milieu (Mosher & Gunderson, 1979). These quality characteristics are difficult to measure and were not investigated in the present evaluation. It is possible that the effect of the bilingual/bicultural milieu is to add to the quality of care directly in proportion to the relevancy of the milieu. Whether the effects of the bilingual/bicultural milieu translate directly into societal payoffs, however, was not addressed in this report but will be addressed in a follow-up report.

Statistically significant improvement in patient's psychiatric functioning and social and work levels was not found in either the experimental or the control group following one month of hospitalization. Some of the reasons for this may perhaps be related to the insensitivity of the measures employed, the short duration of inpatient hospitalization (one month) before collecting the measures, and to the chronicity of the patients. The patients in the study (experimental and control groups combined) were, as a whole, moderately chronic. The average total length of hospitalization for the group was 1.83 years with the average number of previous admissions being 3.4. Most of the patients (79 percent) had been admitted previously. Based on staff ratings, 78 percent of the experimental patients and 68 percent of the control patients were rated as having improved with regard to their primary psychiatric problem at time of discharge; however, gains were small and not statistically significant.

The more acute patients were found to gain most from hospitalization, particularly in the experimental group. Acute patients achieved the greatest improvement in terms of their primary psychiatric and social problems identified at time of admission. The more chronic the patient the less was the improvement seen in psychiatric and social functioning and the longer was the patient's present hospitalization.

The more chronic patients in the study were more likely to function at a lower social and work level than the more acute patients. The more chronic patients were also more likely to be older, need more care, and be more Mexican-oriented in terms of their level of acculturation.

An interesting finding and one that supports the notion of culturally compatible treatment programming relates to level of acculturation and chronicity. The more Mexican-oriented patients were more likely to be chronic and require longer lengths of stay, particularly in the control group. They were also more likely to make greater gains in terms of their primary psychiatric goal in the experimental program. These findings indicate that the experimental program was more effective in treatment for the very Mexican-oriented patient than were the control programs.

The results of the evaluation also add much to our understanding of the role of acculturation in mental illness and its treatment among Mexican-Americans. Level of acculturation was measured on a five-point scale from (1) Mexican; (2) Mexican-oriented bicultural; (3) Syntonic bilingual/bicultural; (4) Anglo-oriented bicultural; to (5) Anglicized. Acculturation level was not found to be correlated with any indicators of severity of psychiatric pathology. Level of acculturation was also not correlated with any of the 12 psychotic factors on the Psychotic Inpatient Profile.

This finding differs from those reported by Fábrega (1970) in which he found that unacculturated Mexican-Americans present clinical features that suggest greater psychoticism. It also appears to differ from Jaco's hypothesis (1957), which predicts that psychoticism in Mexican-Americans will take on a different form based on level of acculturation.

Level of acculturation, however, was found to be related to social and work level functioning. Patients who were more Mexican-oriented were more likely to function at lower social and work levels than were the Anglo-oriented patients. Patients who were more Anglo-oriented, on the other hand, were more likely to function at higher social and work levels. The more Anglo-oriented patients were also more likely to be acute, younger, better educated, and require less medication.

The findings in general support the notion that patients who are functioning better to begin with in terms of social and work levels and amount of care needed and who are more acute benefit the most from hospitalization. These findings and other findings related to the psychotic characteristics of the subjects, and their demographic characteristics, indicate that the sample as a whole was extremely similar to its Anglo counterparts. The psychotic profiles of the Mexican-American patients were well within the norms for psychotic patients in general on the Psychotic Inpatient Profile. The average age of the patients was 34, most were males, most were never married and a large portion were living with their families (62.3).

In summary, Mexican-American patients, particularly those that were more Mexican-oriented, were found to benefit most from the bilingual/bicultural treatment approach. The bilingual/bicultural treatment program was found to be no different from the control programs in terms of producing beneficial psychiatric change. Both the experimental and control programs had difficulty in demonstrating significant psychiatric change following one month of treatment. Staff ratings were found to be more sensitive in depicting behavioral change than were the standardized instruments employed in the study. The experimental treatment program was found to engage its patients in significantly more hours of rehabilitation treatment than the control treatment programs. The bilingual/bicultural treatment milieu of the experimental program was believed to be responsible for a number of quality of care characteristics that facilitate treatment.

For the most part, the patients as a whole were moderately chronic and required on the average approximately three months of treatment prior to discharge. Acute patients were more likely to benefit from hospitalization and from the bilingual/bicultural treatment program. In conclusion, the results of the present evaluation add to the literature by supporting the relevancy of culturally sensitive treatment programming and empirically add to the validity of the concept behind the Bilingual/Bicultural Treatment Program at the San Antonio State Hospital.

REFERENCES

Aumack, L. A social adjustment behavior rating scale. Journal of Clinical Psychology, 1962, 18, 436–41.

Cuéllar, I., Harris, L. C., & Jasso, R. An acculturation rating scale for Mexican American normal and clinical populations. Hispanic Journal of Behavioral Sciences, 1980, 2, No. 3, in press.

Fábrega, H., Jr. Mexican Americans of Texas: Some social psychiatric features. In E. B. Broday (Ed.), Behavior in new environments. Beverly Hills, Calif.: Sage Publications, 1970.

Giordano, J., & Giordano, G. P. Ethnicity and community mental health. Community Mental Health Review, 1976, 1, No. 3, 1–26.

Hollister, L. E. Clinical use of psychotherapeutic drugs. Springfield, Ill.: Charles Thomas, 1973.

Hollingshead, A. B., & Redlich, F. C. Social class and mental illness: A community study. New York: Wiley, 1958.

Jaco, E. Social factors in mental disorders in Texas. Social Problems, 1957, 4, No. 4.

Lorr, M., & Vestre, D. The psychotic inpatient profile: A nurse's observation scale. Journal of Clinical Psychology, 1969, 25, 137–40.

Mosher, L. R., & Gunderson, J. G. Group, family, milieu, and community support systems treatment for schizophrenia. In L. Bellak (Ed.), Disorders of the schizophrenic syndrome. New York: Basic Books, 1979.

Padilla, A. M., Ruiz, A., & Álvarez, R. Community mental health services for the Spanish-speaking surname population. American Psychologist, 1975, 30, 892-905.

Padilla, A. M., & Ruiz, R. A. Latino mental health: A review of the literature (HEW Publication No. HSM 73-9143). Washington, D.C.: U.S. Government Printing Office, 1973.

Rabkin, J. G., & Struening, E. L. Ethnicity, social class and mental illness in New York City: A social area analysis of five ethnic groups. New York: Institute of Pluralism and Group Identity, American Jewish Committee, 1975.

Ramírez, D. G. A review of the literature on the underutilization of mental health services by Mexican Americans: Implications for future research and service delivery. San Antonio, Tex.: Intercultural Development Research Association, 1980.

Report to the President's Commission on Mental Health from the Special Populations Sub-task Panel on Mental Health of Hispanic Americans, Los Angeles: Spanish-Speaking Mental Health Research Center, University of California, Los Angeles, 1978.

Sanua, V. D. Sociocultural aspects of psychotherapy and treatment: A review of the literature. In L. E. Abt & F. Bellak (Eds.), Progress in clinical psychology (Vol. 3). New York: Grune and Stratton, 1966.

Torrey, E. F. The mind game: Witchdoctors and psychiatrists. New York: Emerson Hall, 1972.

10

RESPONDING TO STRESS: ETHNIC AND SEX DIFFERENCES IN COPING BEHAVIOR

A. Patrícia Mendoza

Little is known about the patterns of coping that are effective for university students, especially minority students such as Mexican-Americans. Existing data support the fact that psychological stress is an important factor that is related to higher attrition rates for Mexican-American university students than for their Anglo peers (Cope & Hannah, 1975; Muñoz & Garcia-Bahne, 1978; Vásquez, 1978). Data indicate further that of those Mexican-Americans who do enroll in universities, only one in four actually complete their degree in comparison to one in two Anglos (U.S. Commission on Civil Rights, 1971).

Available literature in the area of stress and coping establishes that there is a wide range of individual differences in response to stress depending on the appraisal of threatening elements in a situation and the significance of these elements to the individual (Coelho, Hamburg, & Adams, 1974; Lazarus, 1978). Coping behavior is a product of this appraisal as well as biologic factors, learning opportunities, and environmental experiences. It is a well-documented fact that not only learning opportunities and environmental experiences but also perceptions of the university setting tend to be different for Chicanos and Anglos (Pitcher & Hanson, 1978; Muñoz & Garcia-Bahne, 1978; Garza & Widlak, 1976; Ramírez & Castañeda, 1974; Guerra, 1970).

While the area of stress has enjoyed extensive investigation since the 1950s, interest in its companion concept, coping, has only recently been manifested. Current stress and coping researchers have recognized that stress itself as a concept is secondary in significance when compared to coping. A coping paradigm advanced by Lazarus (1978) has provided a means to explain the relationship between stress and coping. His theoretical construct, <u>cognitive appraisal</u>, suggests that events in the environment are neutral and do not of themselves produce stress;

it is instead the individual's perception or appraisal of these events that makes them not only stressful to the individual but will also affect the manner in which he/she chooses to cope with the stressful event. The manner in which a person thinks, feels, or acts is a product of the interaction of external situational factors, characteristics of the individual, and the coping responses available to the individual.

The Sources-of-Variance model formulated by Lazarus, Averill and Opton (1974) allows for a simultaneous investigation of these three important variables in stress and coping research (that is, Environmental Situations × Personality Resources × Coping Responses). The primary focus of the present investigation was to determine the efficacy of responses used by Anglo and Mexican-American students to cope with stress they experience in the university setting and secondarily to ascertain the patterns of coping utilized by these students in order to successfully cope with stress.

Differences in level of stress, coping behavior, and personality resources between Anglo and Mexican-American university students were also determined.

METHOD

The sample consisted of a random group of 1,601 University of Texas students chosen from the Spring 1979 computer files and stratified on dimensions of sex, ethnicity, and classification. From this sample, 243 Anglo respondents and 234 Mexican-American respondents (30 percent response rate) were placed in their respective category on the basis of sex (that is, male or female), ethnicity (Anglo or Mexican-American), and classification (Freshman and Senior).

Instrumentation

The absence of an existing instrument that would allow simultaneous measurement of stress, coping, and personality dimensions called for the construction of a special instrument, the Coping Response Inventory (CRI)—College Student Form (Mendoza, 1979). The CRI consists of three subscales (Stress, Interference, and Coping Responses), each included in four domains (Academic, Financial, Familial, and Personal) considered to be problematic for students in higher education (Muñoz & Garcia-Bahne, 1978) and personality dimension scales based on Rosenberg's Self-Esteem Inventory (1965).

DEVELOPMENT OF THE COPING RESPONSE INVENTORY

Lazarus, Averill, & Opton (1974) have constructed the Sources-of-Variance model to account for the identified critical variables in coping research. This model served as a theoretical basis for the construction of an appropriate instrument to assess sources of stress in the environment, responses which are utilized to cope with those stresses, and the personality resources of the individual. In a study that examined the coping styles of graduate students by eliciting their emotional reaction to stressful situations, Kjerluff and Wiggins (1976) concluded that a situational inventory could be developed which could be predictive of adaptive emotional coping in stressful situations encountered in a university setting.

Pearlin and Schooler (1978) utilized a structured interview in their investigation of the structure of coping. Their investigation considered the efficacy of coping responses used by individuals to deal with stress in the various role areas in which they participate. The format utilized in the structured interview provided the format for a paper and pencil instrument used in this study, the Coping Response Inventory. The Sources-of-Variance model (Lazarus, Averill, & Opton, 1974) with an overlay of the Coping Response Inventory (Mendoza, 1979) is presented in Table 10.1.

Stress Scales

Stress was considered to be a measure of emotional upset due to stressful events in the university environment and further operationally defined by the scores obtained on the four domain scales, Academic, Personal, Familial, and Financial, based on the College Environmental Stress Index (CESI) by Muñoz & Garcia-Bahne (1978). The CESI was based on work done by Holmes and Rahe (1967) and emanated from the Life Stress Laboratory at the University of California, San Diego. Two assumptions underlie the construction and use of the CESI: first, perceived stress is the same as actual or experienced stress, and second, subjects will be able to identify the intensity of stress they would experience as a result of specific items. The four stress areas included in this instrument have been identified as areas of concern for students in higher education and correspond to those areas identified by University of Texas students as problematic (Pitcher & Hanson, 1978; Muñoz & Garcia-Bahne, 1978). The procedure of formulating a self-report inventory has been

TABLE 10.1

Sources-of-Variance Model

Coping response inventory	Environmental Demands	×	Personal Characteristic	×	Coping Responses
	Stress Scales		Personality Scales		Coping Scales
	Academic		Self-denigration		Change environment
	Financial		Self-esteem		Change beliefs
	Personal		Mastery		Acceptance/resignation
	Familial				

Source: Compiled by the authors.

suggested as a viable alternative to deal with the complexity of a structured interview while yielding essentially the same data (Bonjean & Vance, 1968).

The CRI (Mendoza, 1979) consists of three types of scales, Stress, Coping, and Interference, which correspond to the variables contained within the Sources-of-Variance model (Lazarus, Averill, & Opton, 1974) and four domains that have been identified as problematic for students in higher education (Muñoz & Garcia-Bahne, 1978), Academic, Financial, Familial, Personal. Students were asked to first, identify the level of stress that they experience as a result of particular stressors in that domain; second, identify level of interference that they experienced as a result of those domain stressors; and third, identify the specific coping responses they use to deal with those stressors. Also included are personality scales that measure self-esteem, self-denigration, and mastery.

Coping Scales

Coping responses were defined by the scores obtained on Likert-type coping scales composed of items reflecting things that people do in their efforts to deal with stress they encounter in the university environment. These items were representative of strategies compiled from an extensive literature review in the area of coping (Coelho, Hamburg, & Murphey, 1963; Gilbert, 1976; Hamburg & Adams, 1967; Lazarus, 1977; Mechanic, 1962; Pearlin & Schooler, 1978; Sidle, Moose, Adams, & Cady, 1969; Silber, Coelho, Murphey, Hamburg, Pearlin, & Rosenberg, 1961a). Additional examples were obtained from responses provided by 12.5 percent of 400 University of Texas students sampled in the Fall of 1978.

The taxonomy of coping formulated by Lazarus (1977) served as a guide for the organization of the coping strategies into categories. Further support for the taxonomy was provided by data obtained by Pearlin and Schooler (1978). There seem to be three major types or categories of coping responses that emerge from these previous formulations:

1. Responses that change the situation out of which strainful experience arises (Lazarus' Direct Action type).
2. Responses that control the meaning of the strainful experience (Lazarus' Intrapsychic Processes type).
3. Responses that function to control stress (Acceptance/Resignation type in Pearlin & Schooler; no corresponding type in Lazarus' taxonomy).

Personality Scales

Personality was obtained on a Likert rating scale based on items derived from Rosenberg's (1965) Self-Esteem Rating Scale that were utilized by Pearlin and Schooler (1978) in their study. Specifically, three personality resources that are related to coping which emerged from that investigation were included for study:

1. Self-Esteem, which was measured by five items indicating the positiveness of one's attitude toward oneself.
2. Self-Denigration, which was measured by items indicating the extent to which one holds negative attitudes toward oneself.
3. Mastery, which was measured by items indicating the extent to which one regards one's life-chances as being under one's control in contrast to being fatalistically ruled.

Reliability of Coping Response Inventory

During the Spring semester (1979) the revised form of the CRI was mailed out to a random group of 1,601 University of Texas at Austin students. From this sample there were 532 respondents to the CRI: 243 Anglos, 234 Mexican-Americans, and a sparse representation of the Black population, 55 Blacks. Data were subjected to reliability analysis. Results on the pilot test version of the CRI yielded Cronbach Alpha coefficients ranging from .78 to .88 on the Stress scales, and from .71 to .88 on the Coping scales. Alpha coefficient for Total Stress was .92 and Total Coping was .95.

Because Interference on the pilot test version of the CRI consisted of only one item, no Alpha coefficient for that scale could be computed. Data from this reliability analysis provided information on items from the other three scales that needed to be deleted from the instrument. After this was done, a subsequent reliability analysis on the revised scales yielded a range of Alpha coefficients on the Stress scales from .79 to .89, with Total Stress being .93. Alpha coefficients on the Coping Scales ranged from .78 to .90, with Total Coping being .95.

Reliability analysis computed on data obtained on the CRI responses from the stratified sample of 532 university students yielded Alpha coefficients on the revised Stress scales of the CRI ranging from .78 to .88, with Total Stress being .92. Alpha coefficients on the expanded Interference scales ranged from .80 to .92, with Total Interference being .93.

Alpha coefficients for the Personality scales indicated the following: Esteem scale, .75; Denigration scale, .74; Mastery scale, .74.

PROCEDURE

Early in the spring of 1979, the Coping Response Inventory (CRI)—College Student Form (Mendoza, 1978) was mailed out to the target group of 1,601 students selected randomly from the computer files at the University of Texas at Austin. A cover letter to the questionnaire explained the purpose of the study and elicited students' participation.

Three weeks after the initial mailout, a postcard reminder was sent out to the nonrespondents, resulting in 2 percent additional responses. Approximately one and one-half weeks later, a second follow-up mailout was sent, including a duplicate CRI, a second cover letter, and consent form.

Design of the Study

The design of the study is a between and within 2 × 2 × 2 × 4 design. Four domains (Academic, Financial, Familial, Personal) comprise the between factors. Ethnicity (Anglo and Mexican-American), sex (male and female), and classification (freshman and senior) comprise the within factors. Data obtained on the CRI was standardized ($\overline{X} = 50$, SD = 20), and means and standard deviations were computed for the eight groups (see Table 10.2). Multivariate Analysis of Variance (Manova) was used to determine if there were differences between the groups on stress, interference, coping, and personality by sex, ethnicity, or classification.

Multiple regression analysis with stepwise technique was also used on the data to determine the relative efficacy of coping responses and personality resources so as to simultaneously determine which of the two was more significant.

RESULTS

Stress

Existing stress literature provided data that led to the formulation of the following hypotheses regarding stress:

TABLE 10.2

Standardized Group Means and Standard Deviations on Stress, Coping (by Domain), and Personality Resources for Eight Groups

	Males								Females							
	Anglo				Mex-Am				Anglo				Mex-Am			
	FR(N=54)		SR(N=61)		FR(N=60)		SR(N=60)		FR(N=77)		SR(N=50)		FR(N=57)		SR(N=57)	
	$\bar{X}$	SD	$\bar{X}$	SD	$\bar{X}$	SD	$\bar{X}$	SD	$\bar{X}$	SD	$\bar{X}$	SD	$\bar{X}$	SD	$\bar{X}$	SD
Academic																
Stress	48.67	9.80	46.31	8.52	50.11	10.31	48.21	10.63	52.17	9.92	49.53	7.79	51.57	10.57	52.90	10.52
Coping	51.10	8.25	49.05	8.64	51.53	9.06	48.53	8.39	54.44	7.43	50.63	7.73	53.41	8.91	48.43	9.07
Interference	48.89	10.39	47.90	9.81	50.15	10.33	49.32	8.79	51.05	9.82	48.63	9.18	50.43	10.44	53.18	10.73
Financial																
Stress	48.19	10.09	46.13	9.13	50.41	9.85	48.49	10.01	50.56	9.58	53.81	8.60	49.19	11.41	53.06	9.68
Coping	51.28	9.38	48.90	10.41	53.33	8.93	48.73	8.97	53.18	7.65	52.81	9.30	53.97	8.00	51.42	6.39
Interference	50.28	8.80	45.72	9.31	50.69	11.43	51.37	8.72	48.25	8.76	51.66	9.82	49.33	10.02	53.73	11.43
Familial																
Stress	50.48	9.68	46.38	9.27	50.15	9.62	45.24	9.07	52.16	10.62	52.33	10.01	51.15	9.98	51.51	9.30
Coping	50.95	8.06	46.30	9.34	50.02	8.74	46.73	6.96	55.58	8.55	54.06	8.74	53.05	7.93	51.15	7.93
Interference	48.68	9.90	47.41	10.86	50.43	10.01	48.16	8.69	52.67	10.71	49.02	8.61	51.51	10.95	51.37	8.76
Personal																
Stress	49.78	10.07	46.64	8.97	50.09	9.17	47.46	9.54	52.48	11.40	51.11	10.22	50.66	8.15	51.39	10.78
Coping	51.26	9.91	48.61	8.21	51.43	7.49	46.81	8.35	54.79	8.25	52.93	9.33	54.05	8.97	49.29	7.76
Interference	51.32	9.32	48.45	8.77	50.08	10.51	47.35	9.18	51.52	10.83	49.77	9.74	50.39	9.47	50.89	11.41
Personality Resources																
Esteem	49.30	9.85	52.98	8.04	49.51	10.75	52.59	7.56	49.85	10.05	47.85	11.49	47.43	11.04	50.11	9.61
Denigration	49.31	10.57	49.58	9.24	49.55	9.87	49.16	9.54	49.97	9.25	50.74	9.32	52.36	11.20	50.00	11.45
Mastery	51.75	10.43	49.14	10.09	49.45	9.82	47.83	9.19	50.74	10.41	49.62	9.50	52.05	9.97	50.24	10.97

Note: Data has been standardized, $\bar{X}$=50 and SD=10.
Source: Compiled by the author.

1. There would be significant differences between Mexican-Americans and Anglos on domain stress, such that Mexican-Americans would obtain higher stress means than Anglos on Financial and Academic domains, with no differences expected in Personal or Familial domains.
2. There would be significant main effect classification differences, such that Freshmen would report higher stress means than Seniors.
3. There would be significant classification by sex interaction effects, such that Senior females would report higher stress levels than Freshmen females or Freshmen and Senior males.
4. There would be a significant sex main effect, such that women would obtain higher stress means on all domains than men.
5. There would be a significant classification by sex by ethnicity interaction effect, such that Freshmen Mexican-American females would obtain highest stress means on all domains than any of the other groups.

Table 10.3 shows the results of the Multivariate Analysis of Variance of Stress by ethnicity, sex, and classification within each domain. An examination of the results of the Manova in Table 10.2 indicates a significant sex main effect ($p = .0001$), with females being higher on all domain measures of stress, and a significant classification main effect ($p = .005$), with freshman higher on stress on all domains except for Financial. A significant sex by classification effect ($p - .025$) showed evidence of the sex and classification main effects.

In general, the expected ethnic differences between Anglo and Mexican-American university students on stress were not obtained. These findings corroborate those of Vásquez (1978) based on Anglo and Chicano persisters and nonpersisters at the University of Texas rather than the findings of Muñoz and Garcia-Bahne (1978) who found significant differences between Anglo and Mexican-American students with Chicanos reporting higher levels of stress and females reporting the highest levels of stress. Given that Muñoz and Garcia-Bahne (1978) included students from various University of California campuses while Vásquez (1978) and the present research involved only one University of Texas campus, the California sample is likely a more representative sample of Chicano students enrolled in California universities than the more homogeneous Texas sample.

Another explanation that can be provided from research (González, 1978; Vásquez, 1978; Muñoz & Garcia-Bahne, 1978)

TABLE 10.3

Manova: Stress by Ethnicity, Sex, and Classification
within Academic, Financial, Familial, and Personal Domains

Source	df	F	p
Ethnicity (E)	4	1.89	.1110
Sex(s)	4	5.93	.0001*
Classification (C)	4	3.68	.0058*
E × S	4	0.93	.4449
E × C	4	0.55	.6967
S × C	4	2.79	.0259*
E × S × C	4	0.24	.9173
Error	466		

*$p \leq .05$
Note: Data standardized within domains: $\bar{x} = 50$, SD = 10.
Source: Compiled by the author.

indicates that significantly higher percentages of Texas women
prefer the term "Chicano" over "Mexican-American" in terms of
identification preference. Viewing oneself as a Chicano tends
to indicate that "one sees oneself as part of the Chicano
movement . . . and that one acknowledges the social, economic
and political problems that confront this community" (Muñoz &
Garcia-Bahne, 1978, p. 91). This difference in identification
preferences between female California university students and
University of Texas females points to some noticeable differences
between these two groups of Mexican-Americans.

The findings that women experienced significantly more
stress than men is consistent with previous epidemiological,
environmental, and coping research which has concluded that
women tend to report more stress than men (Greenley & Mechanic,
1976; King & Walsh, 1972; Pearlin & Schooler, 1978).

That seniors would report higher stress means than freshmen was supported with the exception of relatively high stress
in the Personal domain, with higher stress reported by freshmen
Anglo females. The data substantiate findings by Madrazo-
Peterson and Rodríguez (1978) which support the notion that
as students progress through the university experience and

increase their awareness of campus helping services and facilities, their level of stress seems to increase rather than decrease. This would seem to suggest that students gradually reach the realization that existing campus services may not be adequate to the task of helping them cope with the difficulties they experience, and their stress is exacerbated rather than abated.

In spite of fairly consistent data that report the unavailability of adequate finances and often less adequate academic preparation for minority students (Árce, 1976; Muñoz & Garcia-Bahne, 1978; Pitcher & Hanson, 1978; Westbrook, Mijares, & Roberts, 1978), the present data indicated that rather than ethnicity being an important factor in these domains, it was women across all domains—academic, financial, familial, personal—that obtained the highest stress means of all groups. This finding is not that unexpected given the fact that only recently have attitudes and values in socialization practices altered to encompass the importance of higher education for women, a fact that has existed historically for men.

Coping

While literature on coping was even less available, both data as well as conceptual models in this area provided the basis for the following hypothesis concerning coping:

> There would be a significant ethnicity, sex, and classification main effects on coping, such that
> (a) Anglos would obtain higher means on coping scales than Mexican-American students.
> (b) Females would obtain higher means on coping scales than males.
> (c) Seniors would obtain higher means on coping scales than freshmen.

Table 10.4 displays the results of the Manova of Coping × Sex × Class × Ethnicity. A significant sex main effect (p = .0001) and significant classification main effect (p = .0001) can be noted. Although not statistically significant (p = .08), a slight ethnicity trend can be noted.

In general, not all expected findings regarding coping were obtained. Obtained means on the coping scales did not support the expected significant ethnicity main effect. In fact, there were again no ethnicity main effects or interaction effects noted on coping. Data did corroborate earlier research that

TABLE 10.4

Manova: Coping by Ethnicity, Sex, and Classification
within Academic, Financial, Familial, and Personal Domains

Source	df	F	p
Ethnicity (E)	4	.98	.08
Sex (S)	4	8.97	.0001*
Classification (C)	4	5.13	.0001*
E × S	4	.57	.68
E × C	4	1.79	.13
S × C	4	1.89	.11
E × S × C	4	.12	.98
Error	355		

*$p \leq .05$.
Note: Data standardized with domains: $\bar{x} = 50$, SD = 10.
Source: Compiled by the author.

indicated women tended to do more to cope with stress than males
(Greenley & Mechanic, 1976). The third part of this hypothesis
with respect to classification main effects was not supported in
the expected direction. The highest coping means were obtained
by freshmen and not senior students. While it has been found
that freshmen report significantly greater satisfaction with other
students than do members of other classification groups and
generally tend to be more idealistic and optimistic (Madrazo-
Peterson & Rodríguez, 1978), it is Anglo female freshmen, with
the exception of Mexican-American female freshmen in the financial domain, who tend to use coping responses more frequently
to deal with stress experienced in the academic, familial, and
personal domains.

Interference

Although there were no specific hypotheses related to
differences in interference, this measure was an important part
of the analysis and an integral part of the conceptual model utilized in this research. To understand the relationship between

domain stresses and the level of interference experienced in each domain, the obtained interference scores were also standardized, X = 50 and SD = 10.

A Manova was performed on the resulting standardized means on domain interference to determine differences between groups on this variable. Table 10.5 contains the results of this analysis.

It can be noted that there seem to be significant ethnicity (p = .013), sex (p = .039), and classification (p = .004) main effects on domain interference and a sex X classification interaction effect (p = .005) among groups. These data indicate that Mexican-Americans report higher interference means as a result of experienced domain stress than Anglos, with Mexican-American females reporting the highest interference means of all groups. Results of a post hoc Manova data analysis (the univariate F-test with a significance level of .0125) yielded significant results (F = 7.38, p = .0068), indicating that it is particularly in the financial domain that these differences between the groups are occurring.

Freshmen males obtain higher means than freshmen females and senior males and senior females obtain higher interference

TABLE 10.5

Manova: Interference by Ethnicity, Sex, and Classification within Academic, Financial, Familial, and Personal Domains

Source	df	F	p
Ethnicity(E)	4	3.20	.013*
Sex (S)	4	2.55	.039*
Classification (C)	4	3.92	.004*
E × S	4	0.57	.688
E × C	4	1.12	.350
S × C	4	3.80	.005*
E × S × C	4	2.04	.088
Error	451		

*p ≤ .05.
Note: Data standardized within domains: $\overline{X}$ = 50, SD = 10.
Source: Compiled by the author.

means than freshmen females. The univariate F-test with $(1, 454)$ degrees of freedom, yielded an $F = 8.70$ $(p = .0033)$, indicating this difference between females and males occurs in the familial domain.

While expected ethnic main effects and interaction effects did not seem to emerge on the stress variable, it is interesting to note that this difference did occur at the level of interference among groups. Students identified the amount of emotional stress they experienced as a result of stressors in four domains of the university environment. The sample that responded to these stressful events reported basically similar levels of emotional stress. However, when these data are analyzed to determine the level of interference experienced as a result of those identified stresses, that is, how threatening, challenging, limiting, or constructing these stressors were appraised to be) these ethnic differences did emerge. What this finding suggests is that merely asking individuals to identify how stressful they consider environmental events or situations may not be a sufficient means to get to the fullest understanding of what is stressful to the individual. Interference experienced by the individual seems to be a more sensitive measure of cognitive appraisal.

Although both Anglo- and Mexican-American students report the same level of emotional stress due to environmental factors, the meaning that this emotional stress holds for these two groups seems to be different. Perhaps one way of explaining the higher attrition rate for Mexican-Americans when compared to Anglos is that the former group might view dropping out of college as the most viable coping mechanism available to them to deal with the stress.

Personality Resources

There were two hypotheses generated regarding personality resources:

1. There would be a significant ethnicity × sex interaction effect on the personality resources of self-esteem and mastery, such that
   (a) Mexican-American females would obtain higher means on self-esteem than Anglo females.
   (b) Anglo males would obtain lower means on mastery than any other sex and ethnic group.

2. There would be no significant differences in means obtained on self-denigration scales between the eight groups.

The results of the Manova that tested these hypotheses (shown in Table 10.6) failed to yield any significant main effects or interaction effects between self-esteem, denigration, or mastery by ethnicity, sex, and classification. These data do not corroborate previous findings by González (1978) indicating that Chicano families at the University of Texas at Austin obtained higher scores on self-esteem than Anglo females. These data further do not support findings by Emmite and Díaz-Guerrero (1978) that suggest that Mexican-Americans do not feel they have as much control over their environment as other groups in this society do. Only the hypothesis regarding self-denigration was supported.

These findings suggest that Mexican-Americans who attend the University of Texas at Austin are more like their Anglo counterparts than different from them. The numbers of Mexican-American students in attendance at the University at the time of the study are much lower in comparison to Anglo students, that is, 5,534 Anglo freshmen compared to 268 Mexican-American

TABLE 10.6

Manova: Esteem, Denigration, and Mastery by Ethnicity, Sex, and Classification

Source	df	F	p
Ethnicity (E)	3	.20	.90
Sex (S)	3	1.96	.12
Classification (C)	3	2.32	.07
E × S	3	.89	.45
E × C	3	.62	.60
S × C	3	1.95	.12
E × S × C	3	.69	.56
Error	448		

Note: Based on standardized data, $\bar{x} = 50$, SD = 10.
Source: Compiled by the author.

freshmen and 9,527 Anglo seniors compared to 208 Mexican-American seniors. It would seem that those Mexican Americans who decide to attend the University of Texas would tend to be the brightest and/or the most confident of their abilities to succeed at a large university where they might perceive limited support for their efforts. Also, it is likely that individuals who did respond to the study comprise a select subgroup of the population that was sampled, that is, individuals who are least stressed and could take time to respond to the CRI.

Coping Efficacy

Since there has been only one study that has specifically investigated coping efficacy and coping patterns in a community setting (Pearlin & Schooler, 1978), the data provided by this particular investigation led to the formulation of the following research questions:

1. How does the pattern of specific coping responses in regard to particular domain stresses differ across ethnic, sex, and classification groups?
2. How does the pattern of personality resources in regard to particular domain stresses differ across ethnic, sex, and classification groups?
3. Are coping responses or personality resources more effective in coping with stress in particular domains of the university?

It might be important to reinterate the operational definition of coping efficacy used in this study. Coping efficacy was defined by the extent to which coping responses and personality resources were effective in attenuating the interference in performance in the student role experienced by students as a result of experienced stress in that domain (that is, academic, financial, familial, or personal). In other words, students were considered to effectively cope if, although feeling interference in their performance as a student as a result of stress, they were able to reduce the relationship between stress and interference in the particular domain in question. This relationship is represented by the standardized bivariate regression coefficient.

Table 10.7 contains the summary of the findings that address these research questions. To facilitate discussion, the findings will be summarized according to domain.

Academic Domain

It can be noted from the results of Table 10.7 that only freshmen females, two of the groups that reported among the highest means on academic stress (52.17 for Anglos and 51.57 for Mexican-Americans), were able to effect a reduction in the relationship between domain stress and domain interference. The pattern of coping responses that these two groups utilized was somewhat different. For example, acceptance-resignation, change beliefs, and, to a lesser extent, change environment type of coping responses, in that order, used by Anglo females aided the reduction in the bivariate regression coefficient from .63 to .54. Mexican-American females, on the other hand, seemed to use a combination of personality resources and coping responses to reduce the coefficient between academic stress and academic interference from .51 to .36. For this group, a sense of being in control over their environment and their destiny, together with direct efforts to change the situation that is stress-producing, is most effective. Again, for freshmen females, regardless of ethnicity, it can be noted that the pattern is different. Freshmen females seem to effectively reduce the relationship between academic stress and academic interference via the use of change environment, acceptance/resignation, and the personality resource of mastery. The coefficient of .57 reduces to .45.

Financial Domain

All senior groups, excluding Mexican-American females, are successful in reducing the relationship between financial stress and financial interference by use of change environment type of coping response. Anglo female seniors further reduce this relationship between financial stress and financial interference when mastery is added to the equation. Mexican-American seniors seem to also effect a slightly lower reduction in this relationship as a result of positive self-esteem. Mexican-American female seniors predominantly use change belief and acceptance/resignation types of coping responses. For them the relationship between financial interference and financial stress increases slightly, .52 to .53.

Familial Domain

In this domain, freshmen and senior Anglo males and Mexican-American females are the only groups that successfully cope, that is, are successful in reducing the relationship between familial stress and familial interference. For the Anglo males, the coping response of change beliefs is responsible for the

TABLE 10.7

Summary of Findings on Coping Patterns Utilized by Each Group in Each Domain

Groups	Academic	Financial	Familial	Personal
			Domain	
1 Anglo Male Fr			CR–Change Beliefs	PR–Sel-Denigration CR/PR–Denigr., Esteem Master
2 Anglo Male Sr		CR–Change Enviro. CR/PR–Change Enviro/ Beliefs/Accept	CR–Change Beliefs CR/PR–Change Beliefs/ Denigr/Esteem	
3 Anglo Female Fr	CR–Accept/Beliefs/ Enviro. CR/PR–Accept/Beliefs/ Master			
4 Anglo Female Sr		CR–Change Enviro. CR/PR–Master/Enviro/ Accept		
5 Mex–Am Male Fr				PR–Esteem/Dengr. Master CR/PR–Esteem/Enviro.

204

6 Mex-Am Male Sr	CR-Change Enviro/Accept CR/PR-Change Enviro/Esteem/Accept		PR-Denigr/Esteem/Master
7 Mex-Am Female Fr	CR/PR-Master/Enviro/Accept	CR-Accept/Beliefs/Change Enviro. CR/PR-Accept/Beliefs/Denigr/Enviro.	CR/PR-Master/Esteem/Beliefs
8 Mex-Am Female Sr			CR/PR-Accept/Denigr.
Male Fr			PR-Denigr/Esteem CR/PR-Denigr/Esteem
Male Sr	CR-Change Enviro.	CR/PR-Change Enviro/Denigr.	
Female Fr	CR/PR-Enviro/Accept Mastery		CR/PR-Mastery/Beliefs
Female Sr			

Note: CR-Coping Responses

    Change Environment
    Change Beliefs
    Acceptance/Resignation

PR-Personality Resources

    Self-Esteem
    Self-Denigration
    Mastery

CR/PR-Coping Responses and Personality Resources

    Change Environment
    Change Beliefs
    Acceptance/Resignation
    Self-Esteem
    Self-Denigration
    Mastery

Source: Compiled by the author.

reduction in the relationship from .48 to .37 for freshmen and .48 to .38 for seniors. Anglo senior males further reduce the relationship (.48 to .29) for low self-denigration and high self-esteem are variables in the equation. Freshmen Mexican-American females utilize coping responses that help them cope with stress without being overwhelmed by it (that is, acceptance/resignation type of coping responses) to reduce the relationship between familial stress and familial interference, .49 to .30. When the personality resource of low self-denigration is added to the equation, the relationship lowers from .49 to .29.

It is interesting to note the results that emerge when the groups are collapsed without regard to ethnicity. Male seniors successfully attenuate the relationship between familial stress and familial interference (.47 to .37) as a result of the coping pattern comprised of change environment together with an absence of negative feelings about themselves (or low self-denigration).

Personal Domain

All Mexican-American groups and Anglo male freshmen were successful in reducing the relationship between personal stress and personal interference using mainly personality resources. There seems to be no specific coping pattern that can be noted among the effective coping groups. Freshmen Anglo males and senior Mexican-American males utilize low self-denigration, esteem, and mastery, in that order, to reduce the relationship between personal stress and personal interference (.70 to .52 and .46 to .36 respectively). This order differs from that which Pearlin and Schooler (1978) found to be the most related to effective coping (that is, low self-denigration, mastery, and esteem in that order). Mexican-American freshmen males utilize esteem and low self-denigration to reduce the coefficient between personal stress and personal interference from .45 to .30.

Mexican-American freshmen and senior females used a combination of coping responses and personality resources to successfully reduce the relationship between personal stress and personal interference. Freshmen females used the personality resources of mastery and self-esteem together with the change beliefs type of coping response to successfully attenuate stress and interference. Senior females used acceptance/resignation and the personality resource of self-denigration to reduce the relationship between personal stress and personal interference.

In summary, it seems that a combination of coping responses acceptance/resignation and change beliefs, in that order, are most useful to students in helping them attenuate the relationship between academic stress and academic interference. In the financial domain, the data suggest that the change environment type of coping responses (responses that change directly the situation out of which the interfering experience arises) is the most effective means to reduce the relationship between financial interference and financial stress. The more intrapsychic type of coping responses (that is, change beliefs, acceptance/ resignation) seem to be most effective in helping students reduce the relationship between familial stress and familial interference. Personality resources, not coping responses, are the means by which university students successfully reduced the relationship between personal stress and personal interference. Low self-denigration and positive self-esteem primarily contribute to the attenuation between stress and interference in the personal domain. In academic, financial, and familial domains for all groups, except Mexican-American female freshmen and Anglo female seniors, coping responses seem to be more effective than personality responses.

Coping Patterns

A Multivariate Analysis of Covariance (Mancova) of ethnicity × sex × classification with coping, stress, and interference was conducted on summed stress, interference, and coping scores across domains, producing a single score for each of these variables. Consequently, domain is not examined as a within-group factor. In this analysis, differences among domains or among interaction cells with other independent factors may not be tested. The purpose of this particular analysis is the test of parallelism of regression planes. This analysis was undertaken to address the research question of whether the pattern of effective coping responses is the same across ethnicity, sex, and classification groups. This test was used to indicate whether a single regression equation was appropriate for the groups or if separate equations were necessary. The following result was obtained from this analysis:

F-Statistic for Test of Parallelism of Regression
Hyperplanes = 1.29
$\underline{\text{d.f.}}$ = 42 and 888 $\quad$ $\underline{p}$ < .11

The resulting F-statistic for the test of parallelism of regression hyperplanes (F = 1.29; p = .11) indicated little evidence that separate regression equations were necessary for the ethnic, sex, and classification groups studied in this project.

DISCUSSION

An important previous contribution to this area of research (Pearlin & Schooler, 1978) had found that men clearly had the advantage over women in coping effectively with stress. Data from this present study seem to indicate that while women report more stress and utilize coping responses with more frequency to deal with the stress, they seem to be no less effective than men in dealing with stressful situations in certain domains of the university environment. This conclusion seems to substantiate the finding by Pearlin and Schooler (1978) that patterns of coping usage suggested some differential coping advantage in certain role areas. For example, it seems that some student groups may be successful in coping effectively with certain domain stresses, but it is also apparent that different groups may have unequal success when dealing with domain stress in the same manner.

The literature has been generally devoid of basic ecological information regarding stressors that ordinary people or special subgroups experience, their daily dealings with such stressors, or their patterns of coping. This questionnaire study was an attempt to move research out of the laboratory setting into an environmental setting, namely, a university campus. An attempt was made to obtain descriptive data on sources of stress for university students based on sex, ethnicity, and classification while further obtaining data on their personality resources, coping responses they employ to deal with stress, and the efficacy of both of these mechanisms for these groups.

Because of apparent differences that exist in coping usage and the differences in coping advantages in certain areas, it seems imperative to recognize which student groups are more likely to employ those techniques that provide the most effective results in dealing with university stress. It is likewise imperative to understand better the processes by which individuals utilize or avoid various coping responses and resources so that university student personnel can formulate more appropriate intervention services for their diverse student populations.

REFERENCES

Arce, C. H. Chicanos in higher education. Integrated education 1976, 14 (3), 14-18.

Bonjean, C., & Vance, G. A short form measure of self-actualization. Journal of Applied Behavioral Science, 1968, 4 299-312.

Coelho, G. V., Hamburg, D. A., & Adams, J. E. (Eds.). Coping and adaptation. New York: Basic Books, 1974.

Coelho, G., Hamburg, D., & Murphey, E. Coping strategies in a new learning environment. Archives of General Psychiatry, 1963, 9, 433–43.

Cope, R. G., & Hannah, W. Revolving college doors: The causes and consequences of dropping out, stopping out, and transfering. New York: Wiley-Interscience, 1975.

Emmite, P. L., & Díaz-Guerrero, R. Cross-cultural differences and similarities in coping style, anxiety and success-failure on examinations. Ford Foundation Institutional Grant No. 760-0303, 1978.

Garza, R. T., & Widlak, F. W. Antecedents of Chicano and Anglo student perceptions of the university environment. Journal of College Student Personnel, 1976, 17, No. 4, 295–99.

Gilbert, L. Coping Style Questionnaire. Unpublished, c. 1976.

González, A. M. Psychological characteristics associated with biculturalism among Mexican-American college women. Unpublished Ph.D. dissertation, University of Texas at Austin, 1978.

Greenley, J., & Mechanic, D. Social selection in seeking help for psychological problems. Journal of Health and Social Behavior, 1976, 17, 249–62.

Guerra, M. H. The retention of Mexican American students in higher education with special reference to bicultural and and bilingual problems. In H. S. Johnson & W. J. Hernández (Eds.), Educating the Mexican American. Philadelphia: Judson Press, 1970, pp. 124–44.

Hamburg, D. A., & Adams, J. E. A perspective on coping behavior: Seeking and utilizing information in major transitions. Archives of General Psychiatry, 1967, 17, 277–84.

Holmes, T. H., & Rahe, R. H. The Social Readjustment Rating Scale. Journal of Psychosomatic Research, 1967, 11, 212–18.

King, H., & Walsh, W. B. Change in environmental expectations and perceptions. Journal of College Student Personnel, 1972, 13, 331-37.

Kjerluff, K., & Wiggins, N. H. Graduate student styles for coping with stressful situations. Journal of Educational Psychology, 1976, 68, 247-54.

Lazarus, R. S. Cognitive and coping processes in emotion. In A. Monat & R. S. Lazarus (Eds.), Stress and coping: An anthology. New York: Columbia University Press, 1977.

Lazarus, R. S. The stress and coping paradigm. Paper presented at the Critical Evaluation of Behavioral Paradigms for Psychiatric Science Conference, Gleneden Beach, Oregon, November 3-6, 1978.

Lazarus, R. S., Averill, J. R., & Opton, E. M., Jr. (Eds.). Coping and adaptation. New York: Basic Books, 1974.

Madrazo-Peterson, R., & Rodríguez, M. Minority students' perceptions of a university environment. Journal of College Student Personnel, 1978, 19, 259-67.

Mechanic, D. Students under stress. New York: Free Press, 1962.

Mendoza, P. Coping Response Inventory—college student form. Unpublished manuscript, University of Texas at Austin, 1979.

Muñoz, D., & Garcia-Bahne, B. A study of the Chicano experience in higher education. A final report for the Center for Minority Group Mental Health Programs and the National Institute of Mental Health, Grant No. NN24597-01, University of California, San Diego, 1978.

Pearlin, L. I., & Schooler, C. The structure of coping. Journal of Health and Social Behavior, 1978, 19, 2-21.

Pitcher, G., & Hanson, G. R. Student perceptions of the university environment: A student needs survey. Survey reports published by Dean of Students Office, University of Texas, Austin, Texas, 1978.

Ramírez, M., III, & Castañeda, A. Cultural democracy: Bicognitive development and education. New York: Academic Press, 1974.

Rosenberg, M. Society and the adolescent self-image. Princeton: Princeton University Press, 1965.

Sidle, A., Moose, R. H., Adams, J., & Cady, P. Development of a coping scale. Archives of General Psychiatry, 1969, 20, 225-32.

Silber, E., Coelho, G. V., Murphey, E., Hamburg, D., Pearlin, L., & Rosenberg, M. Competent adolescents coping with college decisions. Archives of General Psychiatry, 1961, 5, 517-27. (a)

U.S. Commission on Civil Rights. Mexican-American education study, Report II. The unfinished education: Outcomes for minorities in the five southwestern states. Washington, D.C.: U.S. Government Printing Office, 1971.

Vásquez, M. J. Chicano and Anglo university women: Factors related to their performance, persistence and attrition. Unpublished Ph.D. dissertation. University of Texas at Austin, 1978.

Westbrook, F. D., Mijares, J., & Roberts, J. H. Perceived problem areas by black and white students and hints about comparative counseling needs. Journal of Counseling Psychology, 1978, 25 (2), 119-23.

AUTHOR INDEX

SUBJECT INDEX

acculturation: effects on college students' concerns, 135; empirical application of inclusive model, 77–79; exclusive model of, 76–77; factors affecting acculturation, 72–73; inclusive model of, 73–75; measurement of, 71; treatment outcome of psychiatric inpatients, 179; type versus degree of, 72
Acculturation Rating Scale for Mexican Americans (ARSMA), 170, 179
aptitude tests: anxiety, 98–99; effects of language on, 93; prior coursework, 93–94; short-term instruction, 94–96; test accuracy, 89–92; test speededness, 99–102; testwiseness, 96–97

bilingual/bicultural hospital treatment program (see San Antonio State Hospital)

cognitive style, 77–79
college admission models, 109–11; academic prediction, 111; alternate admissions systems, 111–12; experiments with alternate admissions, 113–17
coping behavior and stress (see stress and coping behavior)
Coping Response Inventory (CRI), 188–89

critical incident technique, 114–15 (see also college admission models)
cultural incorporation, resistance, shift, and transmutation, 74

elderly: health-related variables and work history, 31–32; health status, 30–31; morale and mental health, 38–41; perceptions of aging, 37–38; poverty, 33; sex differences, 32; support systems, 34–37
extended family, 8–15 (see also family)

family: composition and size, 4–5; exchange relationships, 16–17; extended family and familism, 8–15; fertility and child rearing, 6–7; gender roles, 17–19; machismo, 21–23; male dominance and conjugal decision making, 19–21; marriage patterns, 5–6; socioeconomic factors, 7–8

gerontology (see elderly)
Graduate Record Examinations (GRE), 85

hembrismo, 51, 60 (see also family)

machismo, 21–23, 50, 59–60 (see also family)

221

ABOUT THE EDITOR AND CONTRIBUTORS

AUGUSTINE BARÓN, JR., Psy.D., is Program Director for Group Services at the Counseling-Psychological Services Center at the University of Texas in Austin. His Psy.D. dissertation has been published as a monograph entitled The Utilization of Mental Health Services by Mexican-Americans: A Critical Analysis.

He is a licensed psychologist in the state of Texas and received his Psy.D. and Master's degrees in clinical psychology from the University of Illinois at Urbana-Champaign, where he was a Ford Foundation Fellow. Dr. Barón completed a predoctoral internship in clinical psychology at the Fort Logan Mental Health Center in Denver, Colorado, and received his B.A. in psychology, magna cum laude, from Loyola University in New Orleans.

CARLOS H. ÁRCE, Ph.D., is Project Director of the National Chicano Research Network based at the Institute for Social Research, University of Michigan at Ann Arbor. His current research interest is focused on dimensions of Chicano familism and familial identification.

ISRAEL CUÉLLAR, Ph.D., is Director of the Bilingual/ Bicultural Treatment Unit at the San Antonio State Hospital, San Antonio, Texas. He is the coauthor (with L. Harris, and R. Jasso) of "An Acculturation Rating Scale for Mexican American Normal and Clinical Populations," which appeared in the Hispanic Journal of Behavioral Sciences.

ANNA M. GONZÁLEZ, Ph.D., is Assistant Professor of Psychology at Colorado State University in Fort Collins. Her Ph.D. dissertation research was an investigation of the psychological characteristics associated with biculturalism among Mexican-American college women.

LORWEN C. HARRIS, M.A., is a doctoral student in community psychology at the University of Texas at Austin. She is the codeveloper of an acculturation rating scale for Chicanos with I. Cuéllar and R. Jasso.

STEVEN LÓPEZ, M.A., is a doctoral candidate in clinical psychology at the University of California at Los Angeles. He is the author of "Clinical Stereotypes of the Mexican-American" in Chicano Psychology.

JOE L. MARTÍNEZ, Ph.D., is Associate Research Psychologist in the Department of Psychobiology at the University of California at Irvine. He is the editor of Chicano Psychology.

A. PATRÍCIA MENDOZA, Ph.D., is a staff psychologist with the Austin Independent School District in Austin, Texas. Her doctoral research concerned ethnic differences in stress and coping responses.

RICHARD H. MENDOZA, Ph.D., is on the staff of the Laboratory of Comparative Human Cognition at the University of California at San Diego. His Ph.D. dissertation was a cross-cultural study of information-processing styles.

NANCY NARON, M.A., is an Administrative Assistant for the Culture Simulator Project at the Worden School of Social Service, Our Lady of the Lake University, San Antonio, Texas.

FRANK COTA-ROBLES NEWTON, Ph.D., is Project Director of the Multi-Purpose Senior Services Project sponsored by the East Los Angeles Health Task Force in California. He is the coauthor (with R. A. Ruiz) of "Chicano Culture and Mental Health Among the Elderly" in Chicano Aging and Mental Health.

OSCAR RAMÍREZ, Ph.D., is an Assistant Professor in the Department of Psychiatry at the University of Texas Health Sciences Center in San Antonio. His doctoral research analyzed extended family phenomena and mental health among urban Chicanos.

EDWARD T. RINCÓN, Ph.D., is Research Coordinator of the Hispanic Youth Employment Research Center sponsored by the National Council for La Raza in Washington, D.C. His doctoral research studied ethnic differences in test anxiety and performance as a function of test speededness.

JUDE VALDEZ, Ph.D., is Associate Professor of Management and Director of the Center for Economic Development in the College of Business Administration, University of Texas at San Antonio. He is a former Assistant Dean of the College of Liberal Arts at the University of Texas at Austin.